SEXOLOGY RESEARCH AND ISSUES

PAINFUL SEX ASSOCIATED WITH MENOPAUSE

INTERPRETING FDA WARNINGS WHEN CHOOSING A TREATMENT FOR DYSPAREUNIA

SEXOLOGY RESEARCH AND ISSUES

Additional books in this series can be found on Nova's website
under the Series tab.

Additional e-books in this series can be found on Nova's website
under the e-book tab.

SEXOLOGY RESEARCH AND ISSUES

PAINFUL SEX ASSOCIATED WITH MENOPAUSE

INTERPRETING FDA WARNINGS WHEN CHOOSING A TREATMENT FOR DYSPAREUNIA

MICHAEL W. DEGREGORIO
TIMOTHY B. CADMAN
AND
GREGORY T. WURZ

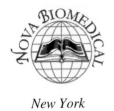

New York

Library of Congress Cataloging-in-Publication Data

ISBN: 978-1-63321-929-8

Library of Congress Control Number: 2014948900

Published by Nova Science Publishers, Inc. † *New York*

Contents

About the Authors

Michael W. DeGregorio has been involved in hormonal research since the early 1980s, including the development of toremifene for the treatment of breast cancer, the study of tamoxifen as a chemopreventive agent, and he was a co-inventor of ospemifene for osteoporosis and menopausal symptoms. He has over 100 scientific publications and is co-author of the book *Tamoxifen and Breast Cancer* (Yale University Press, 1994). Dr. DeGregorio is currently a Professor of Medicine at the University of California, Davis in the Department of Internal Medicine, Division of Hematology and Oncology.

Timothy B. Cadman began his career in clinical pharmacology at Yale University in 1988 and later received an M.B.A. from the University of Oregon in 1999. As a student, he was one of the first to develop analytical methodologies for ospemifene while in Dr. DeGregorio's laboratory. During the past 26 years, Mr. Cadman has been instrumental in critical steps along the ospemifene development pathway. Currently, he continues in his role as a strategic leader in furthering the field of hormonal research at the University of California, Davis in the Department of Internal Medicine, Division of Hematology and Oncology.

Gregory T. Wurz received his B.S. from the University of Texas at San Antonio in 1991 and his doctorate in Pharmacology and Toxicology from the University of California, Davis in 2007. He has published over 40 peer-reviewed research articles, many of which examined the pharmacology of ospemifene. His doctoral dissertation explored ospemifene activity as a breast cancer chemopreventive agent. He has been working with Dr. Michael DeGregorio for 23 years. Dr. Wurz is currently a senior scientist at the University of California, Davis in the Department of Internal Medicine, Division of Hematology and Oncology.

Preface

The most common treatment for menopause-related health issues has been to replace the lost levels of naturally occurring estrogen hormone in a woman's body as she ages. This is called hormone replacement therapy (HRT), and the lead product for this type of treatment is Premarin®, which was first approved for use by the U.S. Food and Drug Administration (FDA) back in 1942. Premarin® is also known as conjugated equine estrogens (CEE) because it is a mixture of estrogens derived from the urine of pregnant horses. Prior to 1962, FDA approval for prescription treatments required merely a demonstration of short-term safety, and thus Premarin® was never subjected to today's rigorous FDA standards, not the least of which requires that all active ingredients of a medication must be defined. Premarin® contains 11 defined compounds and up to 219 additional compounds that have not been defined. Over time, significant health issues have been linked to the long-term use of Premarin® in some patients. Due to increasing concern for public health, the FDA announced in 1997 that approvals for generic forms of Premarin® would no longer be issued.

Dyspareunia is a medical term for painful sexual intercourse that results from vulvar and vaginal atrophy (VVA), which is a common health issue that many women experience during the perimenopausal and postmenopausal stages of life. Until recently, Premarin® had been the only therapy approved by the FDA for the treatment of dyspareunia. In 2013, a new option arrived for women suffering from this health problem. Ospemifene, sold under the trade name Osphena™, is a *non-estrogen* therapy that has been approved by the FDA under today's most rigorous standards. To date, clinical studies have shown that Osphena™ is a safe alternative to Premarin® with fewer risks and more tolerable side effects following short-course (12-week) therapy. While the long-term impacts of Osphena™ still need to be proven, thousands of women have already benefitted from this treatment over years of carefully controlled clinical trials to ensure that it is safe and effective for postmenopausal women. Even though clinical data suggest that Osphena™ is a safe alternative to Premarin® and other estrogen therapies, the FDA has elected to label Osphena™ with health warnings similar to Premarin®, warnings that we believe to be unjustified based on the available data. Osphena™ contains a single, defined, active ingredient that is a non-estrogen. Premarin® is a mixture of 11 known estrogens and up to 219 other compounds with unclear effects on humans. In our opinion, the risks of Osphena™ cannot practically be considered similar to the risks of Premarin®.

The development of Osphena™ was initially based on a public need for safer alternatives for preventing osteoporosis, breast cancer, and other menopausal health issues. Although Osphena™ currently represents a small step towards the achievement of these lofty goals, further research is ongoing in this field of science. The authors of this book have been involved in the study of women's health issues as far back as the 1980s, and we are continuing with our research to this day. The goal of this book is to educate you specifically concerning options for treating dyspareunia. We attempt to present a balanced discussion of estrogen and non-estrogen therapies, but we expect that some readers might conclude that our opinions are biased due to our involvement in the discovery and development of Osphena™. We believe that it is essential to express our opinions as informed scientists, and wherever possible we also include facts and references so that you may draw your own conclusions or discuss them with your doctor. We chose to present you with a question-and-answer style discussion of dyspareunia, including its impact on quality of life and options for treatment. From discovery through FDA approval and beyond, we provide a history of dyspareunia therapies with an emphasis on Premarin® and Osphena™.

Health warnings are commonly misunderstood, sometimes underappreciated and other times overblown. Today's television commercials for FDA-approved medications can be both confusing and overwhelming. In this book, we take the time to review the latest advertisements for Premarin® and Osphena™, explaining all of the stated contraindications, risks, and side effects of these two treatment options. We also provide an education on "boxed warnings" and walk through "package inserts" which are the fine print warnings that come with every prescription. In addition, we provide an update on the latest scientific results of potential breakthroughs for the prevention of osteoporosis and breast cancer that non-estrogen therapies might offer.

We hope that this book will improve your awareness of dyspareunia, help you understand what treatments are available, and guide you through the process of selecting the best option for yourself.

Michael W. DeGregorio
Timothy B. Cadman
Gregory T. Wurz

July 31, 2014

Quality of Life Impacts of Vulvar and Vaginal Atrophy (VVA) and Other Menopausal Symptoms

Abstract

The menopausal transition is a significant time period in a woman's life, marking the end of her reproductive years. Today, the average woman may live one-third or more of her life in postmenopause. Beginning during the menopausal transition (perimenopause) and continuing into postmenopause, women experience a number of different symptoms such as hot flashes and night sweats, insomnia, vulvar and vaginal atrophy (VVA), vaginal dryness, and painful sexual intercourse, known as dyspareunia, any or all of which can negatively affect their quality of life. Although the menopausal symptoms experienced can vary from woman to woman depending on ethnicity, geographic distribution, body mass and other factors, the most characteristic and problematic symptoms of the menopausal transition are hot flashes, or flushes, and night sweats, which are collectively termed vasomotor symptoms, and they are experienced by up to 80% of menopausal women at some point in their lives. These symptoms are a natural result of the declining sex hormone levels seen in women as they progress through perimenopause and into postmenopause. Unlike vasomotor symptoms, which typically decrease in severity and frequency with time, other postmenopausal conditions like VVA and bone loss, known as osteoporosis, are usually chronic and progressive without treatment. Using a question and answer format, this Chapter provides a discussion of the most commonly encountered symptoms experienced by women as they enter the menopausal transition, why they occur, and the potentially negative impacts they may have on health and quality of life.

Introduction

With lifespans increasing throughout the developed world, women can be expected to live approximately one-third of their lives after the menopausal transition. A woman is considered to be in menopause, also termed postmenopause, once she has gone 12 consecutive months since her last menstrual period [1]. In the United States, women reach menopause at an average age of approximately 51 years, but ages can range from as young as 38 years up to 55 years [1]. In 2001, the Stages of Reproductive Aging Workshop (STRAW) designed a staging system, since updated in 2011, to classify reproductive aging in women from their reproductive years through postmenopause [2]. The nomenclature and time periods proposed by STRAW as they relate to perimenopause and postmenopause are used here. Prior to menopause, women progress through what is known as the menopausal transition, also known as perimenopause, which is a time period that may last four or more years. During early perimenopause, women continue to experience monthly menstrual periods, but they begin to vary in length by at least seven days in consecutive cycles. In late perimenopause, which can last up to three years, women may experience episodes of amenorrhea, or cessation of menstrual bleeding, lasting 60 days or more. Perimenopause is characterized by fluctuating levels of the sex hormone estrogen [3] and declining levels of the hormones progesterone and testosterone [1]. It is during late perimenopause and early postmenopause that women are most likely to experience hot flashes and night sweats, which are collectively known as vasomotor symptoms (VMS) [4]. Heart palpitations, or a sensation that the heart is racing, can accompany VMS episodes. During this time frame, women may also begin experiencing the symptoms of vulvar and vaginal atrophy (VVA), namely painful sexual intercourse, or dyspareunia, and vaginal dryness, which typically worsen without treatment as women progress into late postmenopause [5].

Common menopausal symptoms experienced by women as they transition from perimenopause and into menopause—vasomotor symptoms, vaginal dryness and dyspareunia, as mentioned—can negatively impact their quality of life. All of these symptoms result from the naturally declining levels of the female sex hormones estrogen and progesterone as women transition from perimenopause into menopause. While some of these symptoms, such as hot flashes, gradually abate over time, others such as vulvar and vaginal atrophy and osteoporosis, or bone loss, are normally chronic and progressive in some postmenopausal women. It is estimated that as many as 50% of postmenopausal women suffer from vulvar and vaginal atrophy and dyspareunia [6, 7], but many women may be reluctant to seek treatment for these conditions due to cultural and religious differences, social embarrassment or the belief that their symptoms are just a natural consequence of aging that should be accepted [8]. Many women may also simply be unaware that their condition is treatable, and as a result, dyspareunia is often underreported to their doctors [9-11]. Until the early 2000s, the most commonly used remedy to alleviate these symptoms was estrogen replacement therapy in hysterectomized women, or women without a uterus, and hormone replacement therapy (HRT), which contains estrogen combined with the hormone progesterone, in postmenopausal women with a uterus. Following publication of the results of the Heart Estrogen/progestin Replacement Study (HERS) in 1998 [12] and the HERS II [13] and Women's Health Initiative (WHI) estrogen plus progestin trials in 2002 [14], the use of systemic hormone replacement therapy declined markedly [15]. For the treatment of menopausal symptoms such as vulvar and vaginal atrophy in symptomatic women, non-hormonal lubricants and moisturizers and low-dose vaginal estrogen therapy are now the norm [5]. The use of hormone replacement therapy for the treatment of menopausal symptoms and the associated risks are discussed in detail in Chapter 3.

1. What Hormonal Changes Occur During the Menopausal Transition?

Menopause is primarily characterized by a decline in the principal female sex hormone estrogen, also referred to as estradiol. As levels of estrogen begin to fluctuate during perimenopause, many women begin to experience vasomotor symptoms, discussed below. Estrogen levels begin to steadily decline following the last menstrual period, and this can lead to the eventual development of vulvar and vaginal atrophy and osteoporosis (bone loss), which are usually chronic and progressive without treatment. However, changes in other sex hormones also occur during the menopausal transition that can have important consequences. For example, concentrations of progesterone, sometimes referred to as the "pregnancy hormone" due to high levels seen during pregnancy, steadily decline beginning in perimenopause and continuing into postmenopause. Progesterone deficiency can lead to fluid retention, insomnia and irritability, among other symptoms [1]. The principal male sex hormone, testosterone, is also important in normal female sexual function, and as levels of this hormone steadily decline during the menopausal transition, women may experience decreased sexual libido, reduced muscle strength, depression and anxiety [16]. Testosterone is also important in maintaining bladder and urethral musculature, which is the muscle lining the urethra that carries urine out of the bladder [17]. A number of clinical studies in menopausal women have shown improvements in menopausal symptoms and increased sexual desire and satisfaction with the use of testosterone therapy [18-20]. However, the benefits of using testosterone therapy for the treatment of menopausal systems are still unclear. The importance of testosterone in normal female sexual function has been demonstrated in women who became menopausal through surgery, i.e. removal of the ovaries. Because the ovaries normally produce testosterone, these women experience a sharp, approximately 50% decline in testosterone as a result of the surgery [20], and they are significantly more likely to experience reduced sexual desire compared to naturally menopausal women of the same age [21-23].

2. What Are Vasomotor Symptoms (VMS) and Why Do They Happen?

Vasomotor symptoms, i.e. hot flashes and night sweats, are the most characteristic and problematic symptoms associated with menopause [4], affecting 60-80% of perimenopausal and early postmenopausal women [24]. Vasomotor symptoms are so called because they involve the involuntary dilation and constriction, termed vasodilation and vasoconstriction, of the peripheral vasculature, or blood vessels. The dilation and constriction of these blood vessels occurs through the action of the sympathetic ("fight or flight") branch of the autonomic nervous system on the smooth muscles lining the blood vessels. Relaxation of these muscles leads to vessel dilation and increased blood flow into capillary beds, which results in the "flushing" response and sensation of heat during a hot flash episode. Sweat glands are controlled in the same fashion, and sweating episodes often accompany hot flashes. Occasionally, some women experience heart palpitations (i.e. a sensation that the heart is pounding or racing) in combination with hot flash and sweating episodes, particularly at night [25]. In some women, vasomotor symptoms can have a profound impact on quality of life. Fortunately, for some women, these symptoms dissipate within several months [26]; however, the median duration of the period during which vasomotor symptoms are experienced is approximately four years [4, 27], and there are some postmenopausal women who continue to experience these symptoms for 20 years or longer [27].

Although the precise mechanism(s) underlying the occurrence of vasomotor symptoms remains unclear, it is thought that the major cause lies in the part of the brain called the hypothalamus [4, 24], which controls the body's core temperature, among many other critical functions. As estrogen levels fluctuate during perimenopause and steadily decline following the last menstrual period, the normal core body temperature range narrows in symptomatic women such that small increases in core body temperature that are normally innocuous can exceed the upper threshold for heat tolerance [4]. In symptomatic women, these small increases in core body temperature can cause the hypothalamus to trigger a hot flash episode in an attempt to dissipate what the brain perceives as excess heat. Sweating often accompanies the hot flash to increase heat dissipation through evaporative cooling. It has been hypothesized that fluctuating levels of estrogen may lead to changes in the amounts of the neurotransmitters norepinephrine and serotonin in the central nervous system (i.e. the brain and spinal cord), which then leads to flushing and sweating episodes [4, 28, 29]. Neurotransmitters are chemical messengers released by neurons, or brain cells, to transmit signals to other neurons. The administration of estrogen is believed to normalize the production of serotonin and norepinephrine, which then restores normal thermoregulation [4].

This hypothesis is supported by research showing that the administration of non-hormonal agents can alleviate vasomotor symptoms while having no effect on estrogen levels [4]. Furthermore, clonidine, a drug that blocks norepinephrine release, has been shown to increase the sweating threshold in women exhibiting vasomotor symptoms [30], thus reducing these symptoms [31, 32], while yohimbine, a chemical that increases norepinephrine levels, causes hot flash episodes [30]. More recent research on clonidine in symptomatic postmenopausal women compared to asymptomatic women proved to be inconclusive due to a large placebo effect [33], and thus the role of norepinephrine in affecting the reactivity of peripheral blood vessels remains unclear. A placebo is a "fake" medicine (e.g. a sugar pill) given to patients during a clinical study for the purpose of evaluating the psychological effect that may occur simply because a patient thinks she is taking a beneficial medication. Administration of serotonin has generally been shown to have the opposite effect [34, 35]. Interestingly, venlafaxine, a Prozac®-like drug that prevents the re-absorption of serotonin, resulting in increased signaling, causes reduced blood flow to the skin, suggesting that serotonin plays an additional role in the reactions of peripheral blood vessels [36], which is known to be increased in women experiencing vasomotor symptoms. Whether the effects of venlafaxine are mediated centrally (i.e. through the brain) or peripherally (i.e. elsewhere) remains unknown [4]. Paroxetine (Paxil®), another drug that affects the reuptake of serotonin, has also been demonstrated to significantly reduce the incidence of hot flashes [37], which has resulted in the recent FDA approval of low-dose paroxetine for the treatment of moderate to severe hot flashes.

Although vasomotor symptoms affect up to 80% of women at some point in the menopausal transition, not all menopausal women experience these symptoms. It is believed that women who report few or no vasomotor symptom episodes during the menopausal transition have more stable levels of estrogen [1], but there are other factors that can influence the incidence of these symptoms, in addition to racial or ethnic differences. The Study of Women's health Across the Nation (SWAN), which followed 3,302 menopausal women from five different ethnic/racial groups for 10 years, revealed positive associations between vasomotor symptoms and several different genetic, lifestyle and demographic factors, which are discussed in greater detail below. While the significance of these factors varied between the various ethnic/racial groups, the positive associations were common to all groups, meaning that genetics, lifestyle and demographic factors contributed to vasomotor symptoms in all ethnic/racial groups to varying degrees [38]. Despite the involvement of these various factors, the SWAN study showed that menopausal status, the transition to late perimenopause in particular, was the factor most strongly associated with vasomotor symptoms [38].

3. What Triggers Vasomotor Symptom Episodes? Are There Any Risk Factors?

Although vasomotor symptoms can occur at any time, they are often experienced at night. Hot flash episodes can occur spontaneously due to the misperception of excess heat by the brain as discussed above, but they have also been associated with a number of different triggers such as sudden changes in ambient temperature, consumption of caffeinated or alcoholic beverages, stress, embarrassment, or the consumption of any hot beverage [4]. A hot flash typically begins as a sudden sensation of heat in the face and neck area or upper body that radiates downward, sometimes throughout the entire body, followed by flushing and sweating, sometimes profusely [1, 4]. These episodes can last anywhere from about 30 seconds to as long as an hour, but average about 3-4 minutes, and because of this, the term "hot flush" is sometimes preferred over hot flash, which implies a transient event [4]. The North American Menopause Society (NAMS) prefers use of the term "hot flash" [39], and this is the term used throughout this book. As mentioned earlier, it is not uncommon for women to experience heart palpitations during flushing and sweating episodes, especially at night [25], and because of this palpitations are sometimes referred to as a vasomotor symptom.

The SWAN study referenced above is one of the largest community-based, longitudinal studies of the menopausal transition. A longitudinal study is one that follows a set of subjects over a long period of time. With five different ethnic or racial groups—African American, Caucasian (White), Hispanic, Chinese, and Japanese—represented among the 3,302 menopausal women from 42-52 years of age who participated [24, 38], the SWAN study is also one of the most ethnically diverse studies of the menopausal transition. Over the course of more than a decade, this study evaluated the role of reproductive hormones and genetics on vasomotor symptom physiology, the risk factors for vasomotor symptoms, including race or ethnicity, obesity, health behaviors, mood and social and demographic factors, and the associated quality of life symptoms such as sleep disturbances and impaired cognitive function. This study also assessed links between vasomotor symptoms and disease outcomes such as cardiovascular risk and bone health. A wealth of important information on vasomotor symptoms and the menopausal transition was learned in this study.

4. What Are the Main Risk Factors for Vasomotor Symptoms?

Just to reiterate, the single factor most strongly associated with vasomotor symptoms that was identified in the SWAN study is menopausal status. This study did, however, reveal a number of other factors significantly associated with vasomotor symptoms. Among these are lifestyle factors (smoking, obesity), mood (depression, anxiety, stress), demographic factors (race/ethnicity, lower education level) and other factors such as premenstrual symptoms.

4.1. Obesity

Prior to the results of the SWAN study and other large, observational studies of the menopausal transition, it was generally thought that obesity would offer some degree of protection from vasomotor symptoms due to increased levels of circulating estrogen as a result of the conversion of androgens (i.e. male sex hormones) to estrogens in adipose, or fat tissue. However, rather than reducing the incidence of vasomotor symptoms, the SWAN and other studies revealed that obesity, as assessed by body mass index (BMI), may actually be a major risk factor during perimenopause and early postmenopause [24, 40-42]. Body mass index is calculated by dividing one's body weight expressed in kilograms (kg)—one kilogram equals approximately 2.2 pounds—by the square of one's height expressed in meters (m), with one meter being equal to approximately 3.28 feet. A person with a body mass index of 30 kg/m^2 or higher is generally considered to be obese. Even after controlling for other risk factors, body mass index was still significantly associated with vasomotor symptoms. In the SWAN study, women who reported either no or few symptoms had an average body mass index of 28 kg/m^2 compared to an average 31 kg/m^2 in women who reported more frequent symptoms [24].

The association between obesity and vasomotor symptoms may be due to the insulating properties of adipose tissue, which would be consistent with the thermoregulatory model of vasomotor symptoms. However, the relationship between obesity and vasomotor symptoms is not completely understood, and other mechanisms may be involved such as changes in hormone levels [41]. Compared to women with normal body mass index (<25 kg/m^2) during the menopausal transition, obese women were actually found to have lower average estrogen levels, which were associated with an increased probability of experiencing hot flashes. Decreased levels of estrogen in obese women during the menopausal transition may be due to the early onset of ovarian insufficiency (i.e. the ovaries are no longer producing sufficient estrogen), which is not compensated for by the production of estrogen in adipose tissue [41, 43]. These findings are in contrast to studies in postmenopausal women, where obese women were shown to be at a reduced risk of vasomotor symptoms compared to women with normal body mass index [44-46]. Body mass index includes both lean muscle and fat mass, which makes it difficult to determine the relative contribution of fat mass to the risk of vasomotor symptoms. In the SWAN study, an analytical approach used to determine the percentage of body fat showed that a higher percentage of body fat, rather than lean muscle mass, was associated with an increased probability of experiencing vasomotor symptoms after controlling for other factors [47, 48]. Specifically, abdominal fat, and subcutaneous fat (i.e. fat beneath the skin) in particular, was linked to an increased chance of experiencing vasomotor symptoms [48]. Finally, the SWAN study showed that weight gain over time results in an increased risk of developing vasomotor symptoms [49].

4.2. Smoking

Another lifestyle factor that has often been associated with vasomotor symptoms is smoking, and this too was addressed in the SWAN study. To determine the influence of racial/ethnic background on vasomotor symptoms, and whether these differences could be explained by health, lifestyle or other factors, the SWAN study followed a total of 2,784 women over a six-year period [38]. After adjusting for the influence of other factors such as education level and body mass index, smoking was found to significantly increase the overall risk of experiencing vasomotor symptoms by more than 60% compared to nonsmokers. When individual racial/ethnic groups were considered, smoking posed a significant risk of vasomotor symptoms among African Americans and Hispanics [38]. Passive tobacco smoke exposure was also found to be significantly associated with the incidence of vasomotor symptoms, although the duration of exposure did not have a significant impact [42]. It had been previously hypothesized that the link between smoking and vasomotor symptoms was due to the antiestrogenic effects (i.e. estrogen opposing effects) of tobacco smoke [50], but the results of the SWAN study do not support this hypothesis, as estrogen levels measured in this study could not account for the increased risk of vasomotor symptoms due to smoking [42].

4.3. Stress, Depression, and Anxiety

The effects of negative mood, specifically increased stress, depression, and anxiety were found to have a significant negative impact on the probability of experiencing vasomotor symptoms over the six-year follow-up period of the SWAN study. Anxiety in particular was significantly associated with an increased frequency of vasomotor symptoms in all racial/ethnic groups except for Hispanics [38]. Anxiety is well known to be strongly associated with hot flashes [51]. Besides being associated with an increased frequency of vasomotor symptoms, negative mood can also influence the perceived severity of symptoms and even result in increased symptom reporting [24]. In the SWAN study, elevated symptoms of depression were associated with increased odds of experiencing vasomotor symptoms in all racial/ethnic groups, but only Whites and Hispanics showed significantly increased risks

[38]. Despite these results, the connection between negative mood, also known as negative affect, and the occurrence of vasomotor symptoms during the menopausal transition still remains to be elucidated, as both physiological and psychological factors may be involved, not to mention the fact that vasomotor symptoms can have an effect on mood [24].

4.4. Race/Ethnicity and Education

Two other factors found to significantly impact the frequency of vasomotor symptoms during the SWAN study were race/ethnicity and level of education. At the beginning of the study, results showed that African American (46.5%) and Hispanic (49.5%) women were the most likely to report vasomotor symptoms, while Japanese (34.3%) and Chinese (28.9%) women reported the fewest symptoms. Compared to White or Caucasian women (36.6%), the rates of vasomotor symptom reporting for African American and Hispanic women were significantly higher [42]. As the study progressed, African American women consistently reported the most vasomotor symptoms. After a six-year follow-up, African American women reported a 63% higher incidence of vasomotor symptoms, which was significant, compared to Caucasian women after adjusting for other variables [38]. African American women were also the most likely to report their symptoms as bothersome, while Chinese and Japanese women were the least likely compared to Caucasian women [52]. Differences in vasomotor symptom reporting were also seen within racial/ethnic groups. Among Hispanic women in the SWAN study, vasomotor symptom reporting was highest in Central American women and lowest in Cuban women [53]. While these differences in vasomotor symptom reporting between racial/ethnic groups are interesting and remained significant even after controlling for confounding factors such as body mass index and smoking, the underlying reason remains unknown. Non-biological factors such as cultural variation in how vasomotor symptoms are perceived and reported may be at least partially responsible [54].

Another demographic factor found to have a significant impact on the frequency of vasomotor symptoms is level of education. As assessed at the beginning of the SWAN study, women with a college or postgraduate education were less likely to experience vasomotor symptoms while women with less than a high school education or some college were more likely to experience symptoms compared to high school graduates [42]. After six years of follow-up, the prevalence of vasomotor symptoms among women with a high school education or less or some college was significantly greater compared to those women with a postgraduate education. These differences were observed across all racial/ethnic groups except for Hispanics, a group in which uniformity of educational level may have been a contributing factor [38]. Differences in vasomotor symptoms and level of educational attainment persisted even after adjusting for complicating factors such as negative mood, stress, smoking and body mass index, and thus the underlying reason(s) for increased vasomotor symptoms among women with less than a postgraduate education could not be explained [24].

5. How Do Genetics Influence Vasomotor Symptoms?

A number of different studies have examined the links between vasomotor symptoms and alterations in the genes that code for the estrogen receptor as well as the enzymes involved in the synthesis and metabolism of different estrogenic compounds (estradiol, estriol, estrone). The estrogen receptor is a protein that interacts with estrogen to carry out the normal effects of estrogen in a cell. The production of different estrogenic compounds relies on enzymes that convert one hormone into another. These genetic alterations, known as polymorphisms, result in changes in the way different tissues respond to estrogen and changes in how the body makes and breaks down estrogen. The SWAN Genetics Study, which was part of the larger SWAN study and included specimens from 1,538 participants, revealed that alterations in these genes predicted the incidence of vasomotor symptoms among the different racial/ethnic groups involved [55, 56]. Differences in these genes associated with vasomotor symptoms remained even after accounting for confounding factors [24]. Findings obtained from the SWAN Genetics Study are supported by the research of others [57-61]. Collectively, results from the SWAN and other studies suggest that the differences in vasomotor symptoms between the different racial/ethnic groups may be at least partially explained by the variations in genes affecting the activity of estrogen that are inherent in these groups.

6. What Are the Quality of Life Impacts of Vasomotor Symptoms?

6.1. Sleep

The SWAN study evaluated the association between vasomotor symptoms and three major quality of life factors that may be impacted: sleep, mood, and cognitive function, all of which can affect overall health-related quality of life [62]. Several different studies have reported that vasomotor symptoms are strongly associated with perceived sleep disturbance. Likewise, results from the SWAN study showed that vasomotor symptoms, after accounting for other potentially contributing factors, were highly significantly associated with perceived sleep difficulties, including waking up early and the ability to fall asleep and stay asleep [63, 64]. Menopausal status was also significantly associated with difficulty sleeping [64]. A major drawback to these types of studies is that they rely on self-reported sleep disturbance. To address this issue, the SWAN Sleep Study, which included women participating in the core longitudinal study, was designed to include objective measures of sleep patterns in addition to subjective, self-reported sleep symptoms. In contrast to the SWAN core study, results of the sleep study showed that nocturnal vasomotor symptoms were actually associated with better sleep quality, which is consistent with another study showing that while postmenopausal women tend to self-report poorer sleep quality compared to women who are in earlier stages of the menopausal transition, they actually have better sleep quality [65]. Clearly, additional study is needed to adequately address the relationship between vasomotor symptoms and sleep disturbance.

6.2. Mood

The Study of Women's health Across the Nation revealed that negative affect (perceived stress, depression, anxiety) can have a significant impact on the frequency of vasomotor symptoms. However, the relationship between mood and vasomotor symptoms is highly complex, and mood can also be significantly impacted by these symptoms [24]. Results from the SWAN study showed that symptoms of depression and clinical depression were most frequently observed during the period in which vasomotor symptoms were most common, that is, during perimenopause and postmenopause [66-68]. Strengthening the link between vasomotor symptoms and depression, the SWAN and other studies found that perimenopausal women suffering from vasomotor symptoms were at an increased risk of developing depression compared to perimenopausal women not experiencing these symptoms [67, 69, 70]. Several different mechanisms may be responsible for the association between vasomotor symptoms and depression, which can develop simultaneously or one may precede the other [71]. For example, vasomotor symptoms can cause sleep disturbances, which can then lead to depression. On the other hand, because norepinephrine and serotonin activity, which are known to be involved in depression, may also be involved in vasomotor symptoms as discussed earlier, disruptions in these systems may lead to the development of both vasomotor symptoms and depression. It should be pointed out, however, that not all women suffering from vasomotor symptoms develop depression and vice versa, so clearly vasomotor symptoms and depression do not always occur together [24]. Additional study is needed to gain a more complete understanding of the relationship between vasomotor symptoms and depression.

6.3. Cognition

Cognitive impairment, memory problems in particular, is a common complaint among women during the menopausal transition. As estrogen is known to have beneficial effects on brain function [72], changes in this hormone could account for impaired cognitive performance during the menopausal transition [73]. Having vasomotor symptoms appears to impact cognition because women experiencing severe symptoms seem to receive a greater cognitive benefit from hormone therapy than women who are not experiencing severe vasomotor symptoms [74]. The implication is that vasomotor symptoms negatively affect cognition, and a number of studies have addressed this issue. In the SWAN study, an intermittent decline in cognitive performance (processing speed and verbal memory) was seen in perimenopausal women that resolved once these women transitioned to postmenopause [75]. A subsequent analysis showed that the decrease in cognitive performance, specifically learning, could not be accounted for by vasomotor symptoms [73]. Other studies that rely on self-reported vasomotor symptoms agree [76] or conflict with this result [77]. Another study in which vasomotor symptoms were measured objectively showed that they were negatively associated with verbal memory performance [78]. Clearly, the connection between vasomotor symptoms and cognitive impairment during the menopausal transition is controversial, and additional study is needed to further define this association.

7. Are Vasomotor Symptoms Associated with Any Negative Health Consequences?

Vasomotor symptoms have historically been viewed as normal and natural phenomena experienced by women during the menopausal transition and have been assumed to pose no serious health risks beyond typical quality of life issues. Research has begun to reveal, however, that vasomotor symptoms may indeed be associated with some serious, health-related outcomes.

7.1. Cardiovascular Disease

Evidence that cardiovascular disease (CVD) may be associated with vasomotor symptoms began to emerge in large clinical trials of hormone therapy such as the Women's Health Initiative (WHI) and the Heart and Estrogen/progestin Replacement Study (HERS) [79, 80]. In each of these studies, the increased risk of cardiovascular disease with hormone therapy was greatest among those women who reported moderate to severe vasomotor symptoms at study entry. An elevated risk of cardiovascular disease was also seen in older, postmenopausal women experiencing moderate to severe vasomotor symptoms in the WHI observational study [81], which included women suffering from significant vasomotor symptoms who were excluded from the WHI hormone therapy trials. Interestingly, early vasomotor symptoms were associated with a lower risk of cardiovascular disease in the WHI observational study [81]. In agreement with these observations, the SWAN Heart Study, an ancillary study to the SWAN core study, showed that women reporting vasomotor symptoms had poorer outcomes in several measures of cardiovascular disease risk [82-84]. A marker of coronary atherosclerosis, or hardening of the arteries, carotid intima media thickness (i.e. thickness of the neck arteries) was highest among women reporting vasomotor symptoms who were also overweight or obese or who experienced persistent vasomotor symptoms [84]. Given the relationship between vasomotor symptoms and blood vessel function, the association between these symptoms and cardiovascular disease is not surprising. Additional study is needed to determine whether vasomotor symptoms are a symptom of vascular changes that result in cardiovascular disease, or whether moderate to severe vasomotor symptoms lead to the development of cardiovascular disease.

7.2. Bone Turnover and Bone Loss

Osteoporosis, or bone loss, is a chronic condition commonly seen in postmenopausal women. The low level of estrogen after menopause leads to an imbalance in bone formation and bone resorption (i.e. breakdown), collectively known as bone turnover, a loss of bone mineral density, which is a measure of the density of calcium and other minerals in the bone, and weaker more porous bones that have an increased risk of fracture, especially in the hip and spine. Analysis of the data collected between study entry and the fifth annual follow-up visit in the Study of Women's health Across the Nation bone substudy showed that bone mineral density in the spine and hip was significantly lower in those women reporting vasomotor symptoms compared to women without symptoms [85]. To further characterize the association between vasomotor symptoms and bone health in these women, levels of a key indicator of bone turnover in the urine were analyzed in the SWAN bone substudy from baseline to the eighth annual follow-up visit [86]. Results of the urinary indicator analysis showed that early and late perimenopausal women with vasomotor symptoms had a significantly higher rate of bone turnover compared to early and late perimenopausal women without vasomotor symptoms. Among postmenopausal women, those with frequent vasomotor symptoms showed a significantly higher rate of bone turnover compared to postmenopausal women with infrequent symptoms [86]. These differences persisted after controlling for other potentially confounding factors, but follicle-stimulating hormone (FSH) did account for at least some of the association between bone turnover and vasomotor symptoms, and follicle-stimulating hormone has been shown to have direct effects on bone [87]. Follicle-stimulating hormone stimulates the maturation of ovarian follicles, which contain the eggs, and the production of estrogen. Additional study of the links between reduced bone mineral density, bone turnover and vasomotor symptoms is warranted.

8. What Exactly Is Dyspareunia and What Causes It?

Another significant menopausal symptom experienced by women as they progress through the menopausal transition is dyspareunia, or painful sexual intercourse, which is the main focus of this book. Dyspareunia, along with vaginal dryness, itching and incontinence, are the major symptoms of vulvar and vaginal atrophy (VVA), also known as atrophic vaginitis, which is a common condition in postmenopausal women characterized by thinning of the vaginal epithelium, which is the tissue lining the vagina, and atrophy of the vulva, vagina and urinary tract [88]. The symptoms of vulvar and vaginal atrophy are chronic and progressive without treatment in most postmenopausal women, eventually leading to the deterioration of urogenital health and sexual dysfunction [10], which can in turn adversely affect postmenopausal women physically, psychologically and socially [89]. Approximately 60% of postmenopausal women who have never been treated with hormone therapy suffer from vulvar and vaginal atrophy [7, 11, 88], and more than 30% of women who experience dyspareunia and/or vaginal dryness do not report their symptoms to their physicians [88]. These symptoms are a result of the declining estrogen levels seen in perimenopause and postmenopause, which leads to changes in the cells lining the vagina (known as parabasal, intermediate and superficial cells) as well as vaginal pH, which is a measure of the acidity in the vaginal region [6]. One popular measure of vulvar and vaginal atrophy is what is known as the vaginal maturation index (VMI). The vaginal maturation index measures the ratios of the different cell types in the vaginal epithelium. Increases in superficial and intermediate cells and a decrease in parabasal cells indicate an improvement in vulvar and vaginal atrophy. Vaginal pH is normally acidic in premenopausal women, which helps keep microbial growth in check, thereby preventing infection. During the menopausal transition, pH levels begin to increase (become less acidic), which can then lead to an increase in yeast and urinary tract infections [90]. Effective treatment of vulvar and vaginal atrophy, as with either ospemifene or an estrogen-based therapy, leads to a decrease in vaginal pH. Thinning of the vaginal wall, reduced natural lubrication due to vaginal dryness, reduced tissue elasticity and a shortening and narrowing of the vagina can lead to dyspareunia [91].

9. What Impact Do Vaginal Dryness and Dyspareunia Have on Quality of Life?

In the Study of Women's health Across the Nation, approximately 75% of the participants reported that sex was moderately or extremely important, and 78% reported being sexually active at the beginning of the study [92]. Thus vulvar and vaginal atrophy and the associated symptoms of vaginal dryness and dyspareunia can have a significant impact on the sexual health and quality of life of postmenopausal women [11]. As women in the SWAN study progressed through the menopausal transition, sexual desire significantly decreased and vaginal or pelvic pain during intercourse significantly increased. Among the women reporting vaginal dryness on six or more days out of the previous two weeks, dyspareunia was significantly increased and arousal, physical pleasure, and emotional satisfaction were significantly decreased compared to women reporting no vaginal dryness [92]. Despite the prevalence of vulvar and vaginal atrophy and the significant impacts it can have on quality of life among postmenopausal women, this condition is frequently undiagnosed or inadequately treated [7, 93, 94]. Prior to the U.S. Food and Drug Administration (FDA) approval of Osphena™ (ospemifene) in 2013, the only available treatments for vulvar and vaginal atrophy were lubricants and moisturizers, which may bring temporary relief but do nothing to address the underlying condition, or estrogen-based products, which have been associated with a number of potentially serious side effects as discussed in Chapter 3.

Conclusion

As women progress through the menopausal transition, they experience a number of associated symptoms, including hot flashes and night sweats, collectively known as vasomotor symptoms, and vaginal dryness and dyspareunia, which are the main symptoms of vulvar and vaginal atrophy. All of these conditions are a natural consequence of the declining levels of estrogen seen as women transition from perimenopause into postmenopause, and any or all of these symptoms can negatively affect a postmenopausal woman's quality of life. Vasomotor symptoms are the most commonly encountered and problematic symptoms among perimenopausal and early postmenopausal women, but symptoms of vulvar and vaginal atrophy begin to manifest in perimenopause and generally get progressively worse without treatment as women move into postmenopause. In contrast, vasomotor symptoms usually resolve with time. These conditions have traditionally been treated with estrogen-containing products such as Premarin®; however, results of large clinical trials of orally administered hormone replacement therapy have revealed a number of potentially serious side effects, including breast cancer and heart disease. This has led to a reluctance of postmenopausal women to take estrogen-based products, and doctors are now advised to prescribe hormone replacement therapy at the lowest effective dose for the shortest period of time for the treatment of menopausal symptoms. For vulvar and vaginal atrophy, non-hormonal moisturizers and lubricants are now first-line treatment. For the treatment of moderate to severe vulvar and vaginal atrophy that does not respond to lubricants or moisturizers, low-dose oral or vaginally administered estrogen is recommended.

The newest FDA-approved treatment for dyspareunia in postmenopausal women is Osphena™ (ospemifene), which is in a class of drugs known as estrogen receptor agonists/antagonists, a class which includes the breast cancer drugs tamoxifen and toremifene, and the osteoporosis drug raloxifene. These drugs are also commonly referred to as selective estrogen receptor modulators (SERMs). Osphena™ is the first non-estrogen approved for the treatment of moderate to severe dyspareunia, a symptom of vulvar and vaginal atrophy due to menopause, and it has helped satisfy an unmet medical need for safe and effective therapies for vulvar and vaginal atrophy in postmenopausal women who cannot or choose not to take estrogen-based therapies. Two viable therapies for menopausal symptoms are discussed in Chapter 2, and the discovery, development, approval and side effect profiles of conjugated estrogens and Osphena™ are discussed in Chapters 3 and 4, respectively.

References

[1]   Sherif, K. *Hormone Therapy: A Clinical Handbook*. New York: Springer Science+Business Media; 2013. 132 p.

[2]   Harlow, S. D., Gass, M., Hall, J. E., Lobo, R., Maki, P., Rebar, R. W., et al. (2012). Executive summary of the Stages of Reproductive Aging Workshop + 10: addressing the unfinished agenda of staging reproductive aging. *J Clin Endocrinol Metab*, *97(4)*, 1159-1168.

[3]   Tepper, P. G., Randolph, J. F., Jr., McConnell, D. S., Crawford, S. L., El Khoudary, S. R., Joffe, H., et al. (2012). Trajectory clustering of estradiol and follicle-stimulating hormone during the menopausal transition among women in the Study of Women's Health across the Nation (SWAN). *J Clin Endocrinol Metab*, *97(8)*, 2872-2880.

[4]   Archer, D. F., Sturdee, D. W., Baber, R., de Villiers, T. J., Pines, A., Freedman, R. R., et al. (2011). Menopausal hot flushes and night sweats: where are we now? *Climacteric*, *14(5)*, 515-528.

[5]   NAMS (2013). Management of symptomatic vulvovaginal atrophy: 2013 position statement of The North American Menopause Society. *Menopause*, *20(9)*, 888-902.

[6]   Burich, R., DeGregorio, M. (2011). Current treatment options for vulvovaginal atrophy. *Expert Rev Obstet Gynecol*, *6(2)*, 141-151.

[7]   Santoro, N., Komi, J. (2009). Prevalence and impact of vaginal symptoms among postmenopausal women. *J Sex Med*, *6(8)*, 2133-2142.

[8]   Nappi, R. E., Kokot-Kierepa, M. (2010). Women's voices in the menopause: results from an international survey on vaginal atrophy. *Maturitas*, *67(3)*, 233-238.

[9]   Al-Baghdadi, O., Ewies, A. A. (2009). Topical estrogen therapy in the management of postmenopausal vaginal atrophy: an up-to-date overview. *Climacteric*, *12(2)*, 91-105.

[10] Mac Bride, M. B., Rhodes, D. J., Shuster, L. T. (2010). Vulvovaginal atrophy. *Mayo Clin Proc*, *85(1)*, 87-94.

[11] Nappi, R. E., Palacios, S. (2014). Impact of vulvovaginal atrophy on sexual health and quality of life at postmenopause. *Climacteric*, *17(1)*, 3-9.

[12] Hulley, S., Grady, D., Bush, T., Furberg, C., Herrington, D., Riggs, B., et al. (1998). Randomized trial of estrogen plus progestin for secondary prevention of coronary heart disease in postmenopausal women. Heart and Estrogen/progestin Replacement Study (HERS) Research Group. *JAMA*, *280(7)*, 605-613.

[13] Grady, D., Herrington, D., Bittner, V., Blumenthal, R., Davidson, M., Hlatky, M., et al. (2002). Cardiovascular disease outcomes during 6.8 years of hormone therapy: Heart and Estrogen/progestin Replacement Study follow-up (HERS II). *JAMA*, *288(1)*, 49-57.

[14] Rossouw, J. E., Anderson, G. L., Prentice, R. L., LaCroix, A. Z., Kooperberg, C., Stefanick, M. L., et al. (2002). Risks and benefits of estrogen plus progestin in healthy postmenopausal women: principal results From the Women's Health Initiative randomized controlled trial. *JAMA*, *288(3)*, 321-333.

[15] Nappi, R. E., Davis, S. R. (2012). The use of hormone therapy for the maintenance of urogynecological and sexual health post WHI. *Climacteric*, *15(3)*, 267-274.

[16] Lobo, R. A. (2001). Androgens in postmenopausal women: production, possible role, and replacement options. *Obstet Gynecol Surv*, *56(6)*, 361-376.

[17] Sartori, M. G., Feldner, P. C., Jarmy-Di Bella, Z. I., Aquino Castro, R., Baracat, E. C., Rodrigues de Lima, G., et al. (2011). Sexual steroids in urogynecology. *Climacteric*, *14(1)*, 5-14.

[18] Fernandes, T., Costa-Paiva, L. H., Pinto-Neto, A. M. (2014). Efficacy of Vaginally Applied Estrogen, Testosterone, or Polyacrylic Acid on Sexual Function in Postmenopausal Women: A Randomized Controlled Trial. *J Sex Med*;10.1111/jsm.12473.

[19] Glaser, R., York, A. E., Dimitrakakis, C. (2011). Beneficial effects of testosterone therapy in women measured by the validated Menopause Rating Scale (MRS). *Maturitas*, *68(4)*, 355-361.

[20] Hubayter, Z., Simon, J. A. (2008). Testosterone therapy for sexual dysfunction in postmenopausal women. *Climacteric*, *11(3)*, 181-191.

[21] Dennerstein, L., Koochaki, P., Barton, I., Graziottin, A. (2006). Hypoactive sexual desire disorder in menopausal women: a survey of Western European women. *J Sex Med, 3(2)*, 212-222.

[22] Leiblum, S. R., Koochaki, P. E., Rodenberg, C. A., Barton, I. P., Rosen, R. C. (2006). Hypoactive sexual desire disorder in postmenopausal women: US results from the Women's International Study of Health and Sexuality (WISHeS). *Menopause, 13(1)*, 46-56.

[23] Nappi, R. E., Lello, S., Melis, G. B., Albani, F., Polatti, F., Genazzani, A. R. (2009). LEI (Lack of tEstosterone Impact) survey in a clinical sample with surgical menopause. *Climacteric, 12(6)*, 533-540.

[24] Thurston, R. C., Joffe, H. (2011). Vasomotor symptoms and menopause: findings from the Study of Women's Health across the Nation. *Obstet Gynecol Clin North Am, 38(3)*, 489-501.

[25] Freedman, R. R., Kruger, M. L., Wasson, S. L. (2011). Heart rate variability in menopausal hot flashes during sleep. *Menopause, 18(8)*, 897-900.

[26] Nelson, H. D. (2008). Menopause. *Lancet, 371(9614)*, 760-770.

[27] Politi, M. C., Schleinitz, M. D., Col, N. F. (2008). Revisiting the duration of vasomotor symptoms of menopause: a meta-analysis. *J Gen Intern Med, 23(9)*, 1507-1513.

[28] Berendsen, H. H. (2000). The role of serotonin in hot flushes. *Maturitas, 36(3)*, 155-164.

[29] Freedman, R. R. (2005). Pathophysiology and treatment of menopausal hot flashes. *Semin Reprod Med, 23(2)*, 117-125.

[30] Freedman, R. R., Dinsay, R. (2000). Clonidine raises the sweating threshold in symptomatic but not in asymptomatic postmenopausal women. *Fertil Steril, 74(1)*, 20-23.

[31] Goldberg, R. M., Loprinzi, C. L., O'Fallon, J. R., Veeder, M. H., Miser, A. W., Mailliard, J. A., et al. (1994). Transdermal clonidine for ameliorating tamoxifen-induced hot flashes. *J Clin Oncol, 12(1)*, 155-158.

[32] Pandya, K. J., Raubertas, R. F., Flynn, P. J., Hynes, H. E., Rosenbluth, R. J., Kirshner, J. J., et al. (2000). Oral clonidine in postmenopausal patients with breast cancer experiencing tamoxifen-induced hot flashes: a University of Rochester Cancer Center Community Clinical Oncology Program study. *Ann Intern Med, 132(10)*, 788-793.

[33] Sassarini, J., Fox, H., Ferrell, W., Sattar, N., Lumsden, M. A. (2012). Hot flushes, vascular reactivity and the role of the alpha-adrenergic system. *Climacteric, 15(4)*, 332-338.

[34] Clark, W. G., Lipton, J. M. (1986). Changes in body temperature after administration of adrenergic and serotonergic agents and related drugs including antidepressants: II. *Neurosci Biobehav Rev*, *10(2)*, 153-220.

[35] Sipe, K., Leventhal, L., Burroughs, K., Cosmi, S., Johnston, G. H., Deecher, D. C. (2004). Serotonin 2A receptors modulate tail-skin temperature in two rodent models of estrogen deficiency-related thermoregulatory dysfunction. *Brain Res*, *1028(2)*, 191-202.

[36] Sassarini, J., Krishnadas, R., Cavanagh, J., Nicol, A., Pimlott, S. L., Ferrell, W., et al. (2014). Venlafaxine alters microvascular perfusion, [(123)I]-beta-CIT binding and BDI scores in flushing postmenopausal women. *Maturitas*, *77(3)*, 267-273.

[37] Stearns, V., Slack, R., Greep, N., Henry-Tilman, R., Osborne, M., Bunnell, C., et al. (2005). Paroxetine is an effective treatment for hot flashes: results from a prospective randomized clinical trial. *J Clin Oncol*, *23(28)*, 6919-6930.

[38] Gold, E. B., Colvin, A., Avis, N., Bromberger, J., Greendale, G. A., Powell, L., et al. (2006). Longitudinal analysis of the association between vasomotor symptoms and race/ethnicity across the menopausal transition: study of women's health across the nation. *Am J Public Health*, *96(7)*, 1226-1235.

[39] NAMS (2004). Treatment of menopause-associated vasomotor symptoms: position statement of The North American Menopause Society. *Menopause*, *11(1)*, 11-33.

[40] Da Fonseca, A. M., Bagnoli, V. R., Souza, M. A., Azevedo, R. S., Couto Ede, B., Jr., Soares, J. M., Jr., et al. (2013). Impact of age and body mass on the intensity of menopausal symptoms in 5968 Brazilian women. *Gynecol Endocrinol*, *29(2)*, 116-118.

[41] Gallicchio, L., Visvanathan, K., Miller, S. R., Babus, J., Lewis, L. M., Zacur, H., et al. (2005). Body mass, estrogen levels, and hot flashes in midlife women. *Am J Obstet Gynecol*, *193(4)*, 1353-1360.

[42] Gold, E. B., Block, G., Crawford, S., Lachance, L., FitzGerald, G., Miracle, H., et al. (2004). Lifestyle and demographic factors in relation to vasomotor symptoms: baseline results from the Study of Women's Health Across the Nation. *Am J Epidemiol*, *159(12)*, 1189-1199.

[43] Perel, E., Killinger, D. W. (1979). The interconversion and aromatization of androgens by human adipose tissue. *J Steroid Biochem*, *10(6)*, 623-627.

[44] Campagnoli, C., Morra, G., Belforte, P., Belforte, L., Prelato Tousijn, L. (1981). Climacteric symptoms according to body weight in women of different socio-economic groups. *Maturitas, 3(3-4)*, 279-287.

[45] Erlik, Y., Meldrum, D. R., Judd, H. L. (1982). Estrogen levels in postmenopausal women with hot flashes. *Obstet Gynecol, 59(4)*, 403-407.

[46] Sabia, S., Fournier, A., Mesrine, S., Boutron-Ruault, M. C., Clavel-Chapelon, F. (2008). Risk factors for onset of menopausal symptoms: results from a large cohort study. *Maturitas, 60(2)*, 108-121.

[47] Thurston, R. C., Sowers, M. R., Chang, Y., Sternfeld, B., Gold, E. B., Johnston, J. M., et al. (2008). Adiposity and reporting of vasomotor symptoms among midlife women: the study of women's health across the nation. *Am J Epidemiol, 167(1)*, 78-85.

[48] Thurston, R. C., Sowers, M. R., Sutton-Tyrrell, K., Everson-Rose, S. A., Lewis, T. T., Edmundowicz, D., et al. (2008). Abdominal adiposity and hot flashes among midlife women. *Menopause, 15(3)*, 429-434.

[49] Thurston, R. C., Sowers, M. R., Sternfeld, B., Gold, E. B., Bromberger, J., Chang, Y., et al. (2009). Gains in body fat and vasomotor symptom reporting over the menopausal transition: the study of women's health across the nation. *Am J Epidemiol, 170(6)*, 766-774.

[50] Michnovicz, J. J., Hershcopf, R. J., Naganuma, H., Bradlow, H. L., Fishman, J. (1986). Increased 2-hydroxylation of estradiol as a possible mechanism for the anti-estrogenic effect of cigarette smoking. *N Engl J Med, 315(21)*, 1305-1309.

[51] Freeman, E. W., Sammel, M. D., Lin, H., Gracia, C. R., Kapoor, S., Ferdousi, T. (2005). The role of anxiety and hormonal changes in menopausal hot flashes. *Menopause, 12(3)*, 258-266.

[52] Thurston, R. C., Bromberger, J. T., Joffe, H., Avis, N. E., Hess, R., Crandall, C. J., et al. (2008). Beyond frequency: who is most bothered by vasomotor symptoms? *Menopause, 15(5)*, 841-847.

[53] Green, R., Polotsky, A. J., Wildman, R. P., McGinn, A. P., Lin, J., Derby, C., et al. (2010). Menopausal symptoms within a Hispanic cohort: SWAN, the Study of Women's Health Across the Nation. *Climacteric, 13(4)*, 376-384.

[54] Crawford, S. L. (2007). The roles of biologic and nonbiologic factors in cultural differences in vasomotor symptoms measured by surveys. *Menopause, 14(4)*, 725-733.

[55] Crandall, C. J., Crawford, S. L., Gold, E. B. (2006). Vasomotor symptom prevalence is associated with polymorphisms in sex steroid-metabolizing enzymes and receptors. *Am J Med, 119(9 Suppl 1)*, S52-60.

[56] Sowers, M. R., Wilson, A. L., Karvonen-Gutierrez, C. A., Kardia, S. R. (2006). Sex steroid hormone pathway genes and health-related measures in women of 4 races/ethnicities: the Study of Women's Health Across the Nation (SWAN). *Am J Med, 119(9 Suppl 1)*, S103-110.

[57] Malacara, J. M., Perez-Luque, E. L., Martinez-Garza, S., Sanchez-Marin, F. J. (2004). The relationship of estrogen receptor-alpha polymorphism with symptoms and other characteristics in post-menopausal women. *Maturitas, 49(2)*, 163-169.

[58] Rebbeck, T. R., Su, H. I., Sammel, M. D., Lin, H., Tran, T. V., Gracia, C. R., et al. (2010). Effect of hormone metabolism genotypes on steroid hormone levels and menopausal symptoms in a prospective population-based cohort of women experiencing the menopausal transition. *Menopause, 17(5)*, 1026-1034.

[59] Schilling, C., Gallicchio, L., Miller, S. R., Langenberg, P., Zacur, H., Flaws, J. A. (2007). Genetic polymorphisms, hormone levels, and hot flashes in midlife women. *Maturitas, 57(2)*, 120-131.

[60] Visvanathan, K., Gallicchio, L., Schilling, C., Babus, J. K., Lewis, L. M., Miller, S. R., et al. (2005). Cytochrome gene polymorphisms, serum estrogens, and hot flushes in midlife women. *Obstet Gynecol, 106(6)*, 1372-1381.

[61] Woods, N. F., Mitchell, E. S., Tao, Y., Viernes, H. M., Stapleton, P. L., Farin, F. M. (2006). Polymorphisms in the estrogen synthesis and metabolism pathways and symptoms during the menopausal transition: observations from the Seattle Midlife Women's Health Study. *Menopause, 13(6)*, 902-910.

[62] Avis, N. E., Colvin, A., Bromberger, J. T., Hess, R., Matthews, K. A., Ory, M., et al. (2009). Change in health-related quality of life over the menopausal transition in a multiethnic cohort of middle-aged women: Study of Women's Health Across the Nation. *Menopause, 16(5)*, 860-869.

[63] Kravitz, H. M., Ganz, P. A., Bromberger, J., Powell, L. H., Sutton-Tyrrell, K., Meyer, P. M. (2003). Sleep difficulty in women at midlife: a community survey of sleep and the menopausal transition. *Menopause, 10(1)*, 19-28.

[64] Kravitz, H. M., Zhao, X., Bromberger, J. T., Gold, E. B., Hall, M. H., Matthews, K. A., et al. (2008). Sleep disturbance during the menopausal

transition in a multi-ethnic community sample of women. *Sleep*, *31(7)*, 979-990.

[65] Young, T., Rabago, D., Zgierska, A., Austin, D., Laurel, F. (2003). Objective and subjective sleep quality in premenopausal, perimenopausal, and postmenopausal women in the Wisconsin Sleep Cohort Study. *Sleep*, *26(6)*, 667-672.

[66] Bromberger, J. T., Assmann, S. F., Avis, N. E., Schocken, M., Kravitz, H. M., Cordal, A. (2003). Persistent mood symptoms in a multiethnic community cohort of pre- and perimenopausal women. *Am J Epidemiol*, *158(4)*, 347-356.

[67] Bromberger, J. T., Kravitz, H. M., Matthews, K., Youk, A., Brown, C., Feng, W. (2009). Predictors of first lifetime episodes of major depression in midlife women. *Psychol Med*, *39(1)*, 55-64.

[68] Bromberger, J. T., Matthews, K. A., Schott, L. L., Brockwell, S., Avis, N. E., Kravitz, H. M., et al. (2007). Depressive symptoms during the menopausal transition: the Study of Women's Health Across the Nation (SWAN). *J Affect Disord*, *103(1-3)*, 267-272.

[69] Bromberger, J. T., Schott, L. L., Kravitz, H. M., Sowers, M., Avis, N. E., Gold, E. B., et al. (2010). Longitudinal change in reproductive hormones and depressive symptoms across the menopausal transition: results from the Study of Women's Health Across the Nation (SWAN). *Arch Gen Psychiatry*, *67(6)*, 598-607.

[70] Freeman, E. W., Sammel, M. D., Lin, H., Nelson, D. B. (2006). Associations of hormones and menopausal status with depressed mood in women with no history of depression. *Arch Gen Psychiatry*, *63(4)*, 375-382.

[71] Freeman, E. W., Sammel, M. D., Lin, H. (2009). Temporal associations of hot flashes and depression in the transition to menopause. *Menopause*, *16(4)*, 728-734.

[72] Barrett-Connor, E., Laughlin, G. A. (2009). Endogenous and exogenous estrogen, cognitive function, and dementia in postmenopausal women: evidence from epidemiologic studies and clinical trials. *Semin Reprod Med*, *27(3)*, 275-282.

[73] Greendale, G. A., Wight, R. G., Huang, M. H., Avis, N., Gold, E. B., Joffe, H., et al. (2010). Menopause-associated symptoms and cognitive performance: results from the study of women's health across the nation. *Am J Epidemiol*, *171(11)*, 1214-1224.

[74] Maki, P. M., Sundermann, E. (2009). Hormone therapy and cognitive function. *Hum Reprod Update*, *15(6)*, 667-681.

[75] Greendale, G. A., Huang, M. H., Wight, R. G., Seeman, T., Luetters, C., Avis, N. E., et al. (2009). Effects of the menopause transition and hormone use on cognitive performance in midlife women. *Neurology, 72(21)*, 1850-1857.

[76] LeBlanc, E. S., Neiss, M. B., Carello, P. E., Samuels, M. H., Janowsky, J. S. (2007). Hot flashes and estrogen therapy do not influence cognition in early menopausal women. *Menopause, 14(2)*, 191-202.

[77] Joffe, H., Hall, J. E., Gruber, S., Sarmiento, I. A., Cohen, L. S., Yurgelun-Todd, D., et al. (2006). Estrogen therapy selectively enhances prefrontal cognitive processes: a randomized, double-blind, placebo-controlled study with functional magnetic resonance imaging in perimenopausal and recently postmenopausal women. *Menopause, 13(3)*, 411-422.

[78] Maki, P. M., Drogos, L. L., Rubin, L. H., Banuvar, S., Shulman, L. P., Geller, S. E. (2008). Objective hot flashes are negatively related to verbal memory performance in midlife women. *Menopause, 15(5)*, 848-856.

[79] Huang, A. J., Sawaya, G. F., Vittinghoff, E., Lin, F., Grady, D. (2009). Hot flushes, coronary heart disease, and hormone therapy in postmenopausal women. *Menopause, 16(4)*, 639-643.

[80] Rossouw, J. E., Prentice, R. L., Manson, J. E., Wu, L., Barad, D., Barnabei, V. M., et al. (2007). Postmenopausal hormone therapy and risk of cardiovascular disease by age and years since menopause. *JAMA, 297(13)*, 1465-1477.

[81] Szmuilowicz, E. D., Manson, J. E., Rossouw, J. E., Howard, B. V., Margolis, K. L., Greep, N. C., et al. (2011). Vasomotor symptoms and cardiovascular events in postmenopausal women. *Menopause, 18(6)*, 603-610.

[82] Bechlioulis, A., Kalantaridou, S. N., Naka, K. K., Chatzikyriakidou, A., Calis, K. A., Makrigiannakis, A., et al. (2010). Endothelial function, but not carotid intima-media thickness, is affected early in menopause and is associated with severity of hot flushes. *J Clin Endocrinol Metab, 95(3)*, 1199-1206.

[83] Thurston, R. C., Sutton-Tyrrell, K., Everson-Rose, S. A., Hess, R., Matthews, K. A. (2008). Hot flashes and subclinical cardiovascular disease: findings from the Study of Women's Health Across the Nation Heart Study. *Circulation, 118(12)*, 1234-1240.

[84] Thurston, R. C., Sutton-Tyrrell, K., Everson-Rose, S. A., Hess, R., Powell, L. H., Matthews, K. A. (2011). Hot flashes and carotid intima media thickness among midlife women. *Menopause, 18(4)*, 352-358.

[85] Crandall, C. J., Zheng, Y., Crawford, S. L., Thurston, R. C., Gold, E. B., Johnston, J. M., et al. (2009). Presence of vasomotor symptoms is associated with lower bone mineral density: a longitudinal analysis. *Menopause, 16(2)*, 239-246.

[86] Crandall, C. J., Tseng, C. H., Crawford, S. L., Thurston, R. C., Gold, E. B., Johnston, J. M., et al. (2011). Association of menopausal vasomotor symptoms with increased bone turnover during the menopausal transition. *J Bone Miner Res, 26(4)*, 840-849.

[87] Sun, L., Peng, Y., Sharrow, A. C., Iqbal, J., Zhang, Z., Papachristou, D. J., et al. (2006). FSH directly regulates bone mass. *Cell, 125(2)*, 247-260.

[88] Calleja-Agius, J., Brincat, M. P. (2009). Urogenital atrophy. *Climacteric, 12(4)*, 279-285.

[89] Lewis, V. (2009). Undertreatment of menopausal symptoms and novel options for comprehensive management. *Curr Med Res Opin, 25(11)*, 2689-2698.

[90] Lara, L. A., Useche, B., Ferriani, R. A., Reis, R. M., de Sa, M. F., de Freitas, M. M., et al. (2009). The effects of hypoestrogenism on the vaginal wall: interference with the normal sexual response. *J Sex Med, 6(1)*, 30-39.

[91] Goldstein, I., Alexander, J. L. (2005). Practical aspects in the management of vaginal atrophy and sexual dysfunction in perimenopausal and postmenopausal women. *J Sex Med, 2 Suppl 3*, 154-165.

[92] Avis, N. E., Brockwell, S., Randolph, J. F., Jr., Shen, S., Cain, V. S., Ory, M., et al. (2009). Longitudinal changes in sexual functioning as women transition through menopause: results from the Study of Women's Health Across the Nation. *Menopause, 16(3)*, 442-452.

[93] Kingsberg, S. A., Wysocki, S., Magnus, L., Krychman, M. L. (2013). Vulvar and vaginal atrophy in postmenopausal women: findings from the REVIVE (REal Women's VIews of Treatment Options for Menopausal Vaginal ChangEs) survey. *J Sex Med, 10(7)*, 1790-1799.

[94] Nappi, R. E., Kokot-Kierepa, M. (2012). Vaginal Health: Insights, Views & Attitudes (VIVA) - results from an international survey. *Climacteric, 15(1)*, 36-44.

Chapter 2

Interpreting Television Commercials

Abstract

In 2014, television commercial advertisements began to air for two different prescription treatments to address painful intercourse (dyspareunia) caused by menopause. While both Premarin® (conjugated estrogens) Vaginal Cream and Osphena™ (ospemifene) oral tablets have been approved by the U.S. Food and Drug Administration (FDA) specifically for the treatment of moderate to severe painful intercourse associated with vulvar and vaginal atrophy due to menopause, they each take slightly different approaches to marketing themselves. Interestingly, both one-minute advertisements are consumed by at least 30 seconds of safety warnings. In order to comply with FDA regulations and still meet the time constraints of an advertisement, the result has been a minimization of important risk information, a reduction in consumer comprehension, and potentially unwarranted consumer fear of potential side effects. These warnings might be enough to make many suffering women think twice about treating their condition, and that is unfortunate. As an estrogen-based therapy, many long-term studies in humans as well as ongoing monitoring of regular patients have resulted in substantial data to back up the Premarin® warnings. In early 2013, Osphena™ was the first non-estrogen therapy approved by the FDA for the treatment of moderate to severe dyspareunia due to menopause, and appropriate studies have been conducted to ensure that it is a safe and effective therapy. However, because Osphena™ impacts estrogen receptors in the body, the FDA is concerned that it might carry the same long-term risks as estrogen-based therapies. Until long-term studies of Osphena™ are completed and confirmed, the FDA prefers to err on the side of caution and label Osphena™ with contraindications and risks similar to estrogen. There are currently no data to prove that the use of Osphena™ carries the same risks as estrogen. On the contrary, existing data suggest that Osphena™ is safer than estrogen therapies.

Introduction

Television commercial advertisements began to air in 2014 for two different prescription treatments to address painful intercourse (dyspareunia) associated with vulvar and vaginal atrophy (VVA) due to menopause. It should come as no surprise that these treatments are from competing brands—Premarin® (conjugated estrogens) Vaginal Cream and Osphena™ (ospemifene) oral tablets—both claiming to be superior to other treatment options for one reason or another. While both of these treatments have been approved by the U.S. Food and Drug Administration (FDA) specifically for the treatment of moderate to severe painful intercourse, the manufacturers of each of these medications take slightly different approaches to marketing their products. The purpose of this Chapter is to review and compare these two advertisements in order to help you understand how to interpret the messages.

Premarin® (Conjugated Estrogens) Vaginal Cream

Premarin® Vaginal Cream is owned by Wyeth Pharmaceuticals Inc., a subsidiary of Pfizer Inc. In its advertisement [1], you will hear acoustic guitars and other stringed instruments playing a gentle but upbeat melody while the faces of a variety of different postmenopausal women are displayed, initially with looks of concern but soon followed by confident smiles as an off-camera voice explains that Premarin® Vaginal Cream can provide relief for painful intercourse. Words also appear prominently on the screen, with such phrases as "I never expected pain", "rebuild", "it's time", and "there's help". It seems plausible that this text is intended to reinforce the key points of the audio messaging that are heard during the first 35 seconds:

"Nobody told us to expect it. Intercourse that's painful due to menopausal changes. The problem isn't likely to go away on its own. So it's time we do something about it. And there's help... Premarin® Vaginal Cream. A prescription that does what no over-the-counter product was designed to do. It provides estrogens to help rebuild vaginal tissue and makes intercourse more comfortable. Premarin® Vaginal Cream treats vaginal changes due to menopause and moderate to severe pain caused by these changes."

So what is this advertisement really attempting to communicate? First and foremost, we believe that the manufacturer wants postmenopausal women to be aware that painful intercourse due to menopausal changes is not uncommon, but unfortunately it has been a topic of taboo that is not discussed among friends or even with doctors. The manufacturer also appears to want you to realize that this physiological condition will not go away by ignoring it. Therefore, if you are having painful intercourse due to menopause, you can and should do something to reverse the physiological changes and relieve the pain. So why choose Premarin® Vaginal Cream? The manufacturer declares that it literally rebuilds vaginal tissue with regular use and makes intercourse more comfortable. It is true that science backs up these claims [2], and the positive messaging might lead many women to consider Premarin® Vaginal Cream to be just the cure that they need. Then come the next 35 seconds of the advertisement:

"Don't use Premarin® Vaginal Cream if you have had unusual bleeding, breast or uterine cancer, blood clots, liver problems, stroke or heart attack, are allergic to any of its ingredients, or think you're pregnant. Side effects may include headache, pelvic pain, breast pain, vaginal bleeding, and vaginitis. Estrogens may increase your risk of getting cancer of the uterus, strokes, blood clots, or dementia. So use it for the shortest time based on goals and risks. Estrogen should not be used to prevent heart disease, heart attack, stroke, or dementia."

Whoa. Even though happy and confident faces continue to appear on screen during this portion of the messaging, the manufacturer is now telling you that Premarin® Vaginal Cream can actually cause all kinds of serious health problems, it should be avoided by women who have had a history of any number of various ailments, and it should be used for the shortest possible duration. These warnings might be expected to deter many women from trying the treatment, so why would the manufacturer share this information in an advertisement that is intended to encourage its use? The answer is simple. The FDA requires certain prescription drug warnings to be clearly stated in every television advertisement [3]. These FDA regulations regarding direct-to-consumer prescription drug television advertisements were first established in 2007 with the intent to "protect the public health by ensuring that certain high risk and high impact TV ads accurately and effectively communicate key information about advertised products, including their major risks and indications [4]."

Not surprisingly, in February 2014, the FDA issued a request for public comment regarding television advertisement warnings. It has recognized that a one-minute advertisement is frequently consumed by at least 30 seconds of warnings. In order to comply with FDA regulations and still meet the time constraints of an advertisement, the result has been a minimization of important risk information, a reduction in consumer comprehension, and potentially unwarranted consumer fear of potential side effects [5]. A proposed FDA study will investigate the impact of limiting the risks presented in prescription drug television advertisements to those that are serious and actionable, and including a disclosure to alert consumers that there are other product risks not disclosed in the advertisement. However, until FDA regulations are improved, you are forced to take a few extra steps to understand the true risk profile of the prescription treatments that you consider using. More on this topic in a moment.

Osphena™ (Ospemifene) Oral Tablets

Now let's review the television advertisement for Osphena™ oral tablets, owned by Shionogi Inc. [6]. Similar to the Premarin® Vaginal Cream commercial, this one-minute advertisement features confident women and suggestive music. Also like the Premarin® Vaginal Cream advertisement, words prominently appear on the screen, though the phrases are different: "non-estrogen oral pill" and "improves vaginal tissue" are the focus. Clearly, the manufacturer seems to be differentiating Osphena™ oral tablets as a non-topical option free of the side effects of estrogen and with the primary benefit of improving the health of vaginal tissue. These phrases are underlined when the audio messaging is heard during the first 25 seconds:

"If sex is very painful due to menopause, why not do something about it? Ask about Osphena™. For significant relief of painful intercourse due to menopause, Osphena™ is the only non-estrogen oral pill that treats certain physical changes of the vagina, actually improving tissue, which can relieve painful intercourse. Lubricants can't do that. Sex after menopause... it shouldn't have to hurt."

It doesn't take a psychologist to interpret the meaning behind these statements. We believe that Osphena™ has been positioned as a therapy that improves the physiology of vaginal tissue to relieve painful intercourse, and it is better than temporary lubricants because of that.

Can you identify the subtle but important differences between the two advertising campaigns? The manufacturer of Premarin® Vaginal Cream appears to be targeting its product as a *topical cream* therapy that provides *estrogens* to help rebuild vaginal tissue and make intercourse more comfortable, while the manufacturer of Osphena™ seems to be aiming its product as an *oral pill* therapy that provides a *non-estrogen* to rebuild vaginal tissue and make intercourse more comfortable. Is this nothing more than the same result from two different options? Deciding between a cream and an oral pill might be a matter of convenience, but deciding between the use of estrogens and a non-estrogen is an important choice because of the different potential adverse effects. So, how do the adverse effects differ between the two therapies? Well, the next 30 seconds of audio messaging for Osphena™ do have a similar ring to the Premarin® Vaginal Cream advertisement:

"Osphena™ is not for everyone and may increase your risk for uterine cancer, strokes, or blood clots and should not be used in women with these conditions or any of the following: unusual vaginal bleeding, heart attack, severe liver problems, pregnancy, or breast cancer... as it wasn't studied. So talk to your doctor regularly about continuing Osphena™. Call your doctor right away if you have unusual vaginal bleeding, changes in vision or speech, sudden severe headache, leg or chest pain, or shortness of breath. Side effects may include hot flashes, sweating, muscle spasms, and vaginal discharge."

These warnings might be enough to make many suffering women think twice about treating their condition, and that is unfortunate. You can understand the intent of the warnings as required by the FDA, but without a deeper examination of them, it is impossible to understand the likelihood and magnitude of the warnings. So let's take a deeper look at the stated warnings of both Premarin® Vaginal Cream and Osphena™ oral tablets.

As you listen to each of the warnings from the advertisements, they could initially be separated into three groups: contraindications, risks, and side effects. A contraindication is a condition that makes a particular treatment inadvisable, generally because the condition is a possible indication of a greater underlying health issue that could worsen with the introduction of a seemingly unrelated treatment. As an example, if a postmenopausal woman has unusual vaginal bleeding, that could be a symptom of early uterine cancer. Estrogen therapies are known to increase the risk of uterine cancer [7], so anyone with unusual vaginal bleeding could be putting herself at higher risk of promoting an existing uterine cancer if she introduced herself to estrogen therapy. Risks are more straightforward in terms of a warning. Typically, a "risk" is a possible negative health consequence that results from a particular treatment in an otherwise healthy person. Again using estrogen therapy as an example, studies have shown that estrogen increases the risk of developing uterine cancer in women. Therefore uterine cancer is a risk of estrogen therapy [7]. Side effects are typically less concerning than risks. Side effects as described in these advertisements are expected to be "inconveniences" that are temporary in nature, as opposed to risks which have potential long-term health concerns. Now that we understand the three types of warnings, let's compare the advertised warnings of Premarin® Vaginal Cream and Osphena™ oral tablets side-by-side (see Table 2.1).

Table 2.1. Advertisement Warnings

Premarin® Vaginal Cream	Osphena™ Oral Tablets
Contraindications • vaginal bleeding • breast cancer • uterine cancer • heart attack • stroke • blood clots • liver problems • pregnancy • allergic to product ingredients	*Contraindications* • vaginal bleeding • breast cancer • uterine cancer • heart attack • stroke • blood clots • liver problems • pregnancy

Premarin® Vaginal Cream	Osphena™ Oral Tablets
Risks • uterine cancer • stroke • blood clots • dementia	*Risks* • uterine cancer • stroke • blood clots
Side Effects • headache • pelvic pain • breast pain • vaginal bleeding • vaginitis	*Side Effects* • hot flashes • sweating • muscle spasms • vaginal discharge

As you review the list of contraindications and risks, you will notice that they are almost exactly the same for the two therapies. These are two different chemical compounds, one a topical cream and the other an oral tablet, one an estrogen therapy and the other a non-estrogen therapy. How can they have a nearly identical warning profile? Well, this is not a coincidence.

Premarin® (conjugated equine estrogens) was first available to the public in 1942 [8]. Since then, many long-term studies in humans as well as ongoing monitoring of regular patients have resulted in substantial data to back up the Premarin® warnings. In fact, these warnings are found on all estrogen therapies today, including of course Premarin® Vaginal Cream. In contrast, Osphena™ has only been available since 2013. Appropriate studies have been conducted on Osphena™ to ensure that it is a safe and effective therapy, but because it impacts estrogen receptors in the body, the FDA appears concerned that it might carry the same long-term risks as estrogen therapies. There are currently no data to prove that Osphena™ has the same risks as estrogen [9-14]. On the contrary, existing data suggest that Osphena™ is safer than estrogen therapy (see Chapter 4). However, until long-term studies are completed and confirmed, the FDA has chosen to err on the side of caution and label Osphena™ with contraindications and risks similar to estrogen. Dementia is the only risk from Premarin® that has been left off the list of potential Osphena™ risks, which is in and of itself a significant differentiator. However, the extra-cautious approach that the FDA has taken regarding the stated contraindications and risks of Osphena™ might lead you to believe that both Premarin® and Osphena™ have essentially the same risk profile. To reiterate, Premarin® (an estrogen therapy) has been shown to have negative long-term effects as stated in the FDA warnings, but Osphena™ (a non-estrogen therapy) has not been shown to have the same risks.

As you compare the side effects of these two therapies, the differences become more obvious. Premarin® Vaginal Cream can cause some women to experience headaches, pelvic/breast pain, vaginal bleeding, and/or vaginitis. Alternatively, Osphena™ can cause hot flashes, sweating, muscle spasms, and/or vaginal discharge. In both cases, the side effects could be unpleasant if not annoying. However, it seems clear that the two therapies affect the body differently. It is interesting to see that Premarin® Vaginal Cream can actually cause vaginitis (a symptom of which is discomfort during intercourse) when it is being marketed as a treatment for painful intercourse. Nonetheless, it is our opinion that contraindications and risks are the more important warnings to consider when choosing a therapy, and we believe that Osphena™ has a safer risk profile than Premarin®.

In the medical community, Osphena™ is known as a Selective Estrogen Receptor Modulator (SERM), which means that it selectively affects certain tissues that are responsive to estrogen such as bone, breast and vagina. SERMs are also known as estrogen agonists/antagonists because they behave like estrogens in some tissues and like antiestrogens in other tissues. Though Osphena™ is the only SERM approved to treat dyspareunia, other SERMs do exist and have been approved by the FDA for other uses. By definition, SERMs mimic estrogen in some tissues and oppose estrogen in others. In particular, estrogen therapy has been known to cause breast cancer [15], while SERMs are used to fight breast cancer. Tamoxifen (Nolvadex®) has been approved for the treatment of all stages of breast cancer. Toremifene (Fareston®), a SERM closely related to tamoxifen, has also been approved for the treatment of metastatic breast cancer. Selective estrogen receptor modulators have also proven to be very useful for osteoporosis treatment while avoiding the risk of endometrial cancer associated with estrogen treatments [7]. Raloxifene (Evista®) has been FDA approved for the treatment and prevention of postmenopausal osteoporosis. Bazedoxifene, sold under the trade names Conbriza® and Viviant™, while approved only in Europe and Japan for the treatment of postmenopausal osteoporosis, was also approved by the FDA as a combination therapy with Premarin® (Duavee™) for the prevention of postmenopausal osteoporosis and for the treatment of moderate to severe vasomotor symptoms. Chapter 6 provides detailed discussions of the effects of SERMs (tamoxifen, toremifene, raloxifene, bazedoxifene, bazedoxifene/conjugated estrogens and ospemifene) in osteoporosis, and Chapter 7 provides a discussion on the effects of these agents in breast cancer.

As a SERM, Osphena™ acts throughout the body in a manner much more similar to other SERMs than to estrogen. Interestingly, Osphena™ is a major metabolite of toremifene, meaning that Osphena™ is a by-product of toremifene that appears in the body when toremifene is metabolized by the liver. As is the case with many metabolites, Osphena™ has fewer side effects than its parent drug. Because toremifene has been used for *treating* breast cancer for over 15 years, it does not make sense that the FDA has chosen to label Osphena™ as a potential agent for *causing* breast cancer. Actually, as discussed in Chapters 4 and 7, numerous animal studies have shown that Osphena™ is effective in preventing breast cancer, and in some cases treating breast cancer [16]. In addition, toremifene has shown no significant risks of increasing the chances of developing endometrial cancer, cardiovascular disorders, venous thromboembolism, or severe hepatic impairment [17]. To date, Osphena™ has also shown few if any cases of these adverse effects during any of its studies, and any increases compared to placebo were not clinically meaningful. In our opinion, the FDA has been unnecessarily conservative with its decision to require Osphena™ to carry warnings that are more severe than toremifene without data to suggest that the labeled risks could be real.

As already pointed out, raloxifene, sold under the trade name Evista®, is a SERM that has been FDA approved for the treatment and prevention of postmenopausal osteoporosis. In Phase II clinical trials, Osphena™ was compared to raloxifene for its effects on bone turnover, and its efficacy and safety profile were very similar to raloxifene [18]. SERMs are well documented to be safer than pure estrogens, and in our opinion Osphena™ should not be assumed to behave the same as pure estrogens when considering its potential risks. To more fully understand the magnitude of all potential contraindications, risks and side effects of a prescription therapy, the FDA has required a complete disclosure of all safety information in something called a "package insert" which can be found with each prescription.

In Chapter 5, we will review the package insert to help you understand how to interpret all of its information for Premarin® Vaginal Cream and for Osphena™ oral tablets.

Conclusion

Two viable prescription therapies are available today for the treatment of moderate to severe painful intercourse caused by menopause. Premarin® Vaginal Cream is an estrogen therapy that was approved by the FDA in a time when less stringent regulations existed. However, due to Premarin's® long history, its risks are well understood and we believe that this therapy would not be approved under today's FDA standards, which explains why no generic versions of Premarin® have been approved by the FDA. This is discussed in greater detail in the following Chapter. Alternatively, Osphena™ is a non-estrogen therapy that was recently approved under the toughest FDA standards in history and with a more positive safety profile than Premarin®. Only because the FDA is taking an ultra-conservative labeling approach does Osphena™ carry contraindication and risk warnings similar to Premarin®. Osphena™ works in the body differently than estrogens and existing data show that Osphena™ is a safe alternative. However, until time proves that the long-term impacts of Osphena™ are more favorable than Premarin®, postmenopausal women will have to make extra effort to interpret the package insert information that is currently provided with these two prescription therapies.

References

[1]   Pfizer-Inc. Premarin Vaginal Cream. 2014 [cited 2014 June 25, 2014]; Available from: http://www.premarinvaginalcream.com.

[2]   Simon, J. A. (2011). Identifying and treating sexual dysfunction in postmenopausal women: the role of estrogen. *J Womens Health (Larchmt)*, *20(10)*, 1453-1465.

[3]   Lacayo, I. C. FDA to Study Direct-To-Consumer Advertising Warnings Requirements. Weil, Gotshal & Manges LLP; 2014 [cited 2014 June 25, 2014]; Available from: http://product-liability.weil.com/pharmaceutical-law/fda-to-study-direct-to-consumer-advertising-warnings-requirements/.

[4]   U.S.-Food-and-Drug-Administration. Guidance for Industry Direct-to-Consumer Television Advertisements—FDAAA DTC Television Ad Pre-Dissemination Review Program. [PDF]: U.S. Department of Health

and Human Services; 2012 [cited 2014 June 25, 2014]; Available from: http://www.fda.gov/downloads/Drugs/Guidances/UCM295554.pdf.

[5] U.S.-Food-and-Drug-Administration. Agency Information Collection Activities; Proposed Collection; Comment Request; Disclosure Regarding Additional Risks in Direct-to-Consumer Prescription Drug Television Advertisements. Federal Register; 2014 [cited 2014 June 25, 2014]; Available from: https://www.federalregister.gov/articles/ 2014/02/18/2014-03390/agency-information-collection-activities-proposed-collection-comment-request-disclosure-regarding#h-8.

[6] Shionogi-Inc. Osphena. Shionogi Inc.; 2014 [cited 2014 June 25, 2014]; Available from: http://www.osphena.com.

[7] Grady, D., Gebretsadik, T., Kerlikowske, K., Ernster, V., Petitti, D. (1995). Hormone replacement therapy and endometrial cancer risk: a meta-analysis. *Obstet Gynecol, 85(2)*, 304-313.

[8] Stefanick, M. L. (2005). Estrogens and progestins: background and history, trends in use, and guidelines and regimens approved by the US Food and Drug Administration. *Am J Med, 118 Suppl 12B*, 64-73.

[9] Bachmann, G. A., Komi, J. O. (2010). Ospemifene effectively treats vulvovaginal atrophy in postmenopausal women: results from a pivotal phase 3 study. *Menopause, 17(3)*, 480-486.

[10] Goldstein, S. R., Bachmann, G. A., Koninckx, P. R., Lin, V. H., Portman, D. J., Ylikorkala, O. (2014). Ospemifene 12-month safety and efficacy in postmenopausal women with vulvar and vaginal atrophy. *Climacteric, 17(2)*, 173-182.

[11] Portman, D., Palacios, S., Nappi, R. E., Mueck, A. O. (2014). Ospemifene, a non-oestrogen selective oestrogen receptor modulator for the treatment of vaginal dryness associated with postmenopausal vulvar and vaginal atrophy: A randomised, placebo-controlled, phase III trial. *Maturitas, 78(2)*, 91-98.

[12] Portman, D. J., Bachmann, G. A., Simon, J. A. (2013). Ospemifene, a novel selective estrogen receptor modulator for treating dyspareunia associated with postmenopausal vulvar and vaginal atrophy. *Menopause, 20(6)*, 623-630.

[13] Simon, J., Portman, D., Mabey, R. G., Jr. (2014). Long-term safety of ospemifene (52-week extension) in the treatment of vulvar and vaginal atrophy in hysterectomized postmenopausal women. *Maturitas, 77(3)*, 274-281.

[14] Simon, J. A., Lin, V. H., Radovich, C., Bachmann, G. A. (2013). One-year long-term safety extension study of ospemifene for the treatment of

vulvar and vaginal atrophy in postmenopausal women with a uterus. *Menopause, 20(4)*, 418-427.

[15] Rossouw, J. E., Anderson, G. L., Prentice, R. L., LaCroix, A. Z., Kooperberg, C., Stefanick, M. L., et al. (2002). Risks and benefits of estrogen plus progestin in healthy postmenopausal women: principal results From the Women's Health Initiative randomized controlled trial. *JAMA, 288(3)*, 321-333.

[16] Wurz, G. T., Soe, L. H., Degregorio, M. W. (2013). Ospemifene, vulvovaginal atrophy, and breast cancer. *Maturitas, 74(3)*, 220-225.

[17] Fareston® (toremifene citrate) Prescribing Information. Bridgewater, New Jersey: ProStrakan, Inc.; 2012.

[18] Komi, J., Lankinen, K. S., Harkonen, P., DeGregorio, M. W., Voipio, S., Kivinen, S., et al. (2005). Effects of ospemifene and raloxifene on hormonal status, lipids, genital tract, and tolerability in postmenopausal women. *Menopause, 12(2)*, 202-209.

Chapter 3

Premarin®: History and Development of Hormone Replacement Therapy (HRT)

Abstract

The history and development of hormone replacement therapy (HRT), which includes an estrogen, commonly in the form of Premarin® (conjugated equine estrogens or CEE) and a progestin, is indeed interesting. Hormone therapy for menopausal symptoms dates back to the 1890s when a product derived from cow ovaries was introduced. Since then, products derived from the urine of pregnant women were introduced in the early 1930s, followed in the late 1930s by products derived from the urine of pregnant horses, e.g. Premarin®. While a number of other products for the treatment of menopausal symptoms were introduced over the ensuing decades, Premarin®, approved by the U.S. Food and Drug Administration (FDA) in 1942, is still the leading hormone-based product used for the treatment of menopause-related symptoms. This is no coincidence. Prior to 1962, drugs were required to demonstrate only safety, not efficacy, in order to gain FDA approval, and thus Premarin® was never subjected to today's rigorous FDA approval standards, not the least of which is that the active ingredient(s) must be defined. The FDA's Center for Drug Evaluation and Research (CDER) announced in 1997 that approvals for generic forms of Premarin® would no longer be issued, and prior approvals were revoked over bioequivalence, safety and efficacy concerns. This is a result of the fact that, to this day, the active constituents of Premarin® have still not been completely defined, and thus demonstrating that a generic product is bioequivalent to Premarin® is not currently feasible. Therefore, as a result of strict FDA rules to which it was never subjected, the manufacturer of Premarin® has a de facto monopoly on the use of conjugated equine estrogens. The use of estrogen-based products for the treatment of menopausal symptoms steadily increased until 1975, when reports of endometrial cancer led to a dramatic reduction. When the endometrial protective effects of progestins became established, along with the beneficial effects of Premarin® in bone, the use of estrogen products resurged. Controversial reports of reduced coronary heart disease risks with the use of estrogens continued to increase the popularity of these products until 2001. The following year, results of the Women's Health Initiative trial of estrogen plus progestin showed that hormone replacement therapy was associated with increased risks of breast cancer and coronary heart disease, which led to early termination of this trial. Fallout from this trial led to a precipitous decline in the use of hormone replacement therapy and sparked interest in the development of new compounds, e.g. ospemifene, for the treatment of menopausal symptoms.

Introduction

The history of treatment for menopausal symptoms dates back to the 1890s, when one of the first products, Ovarin, was introduced. This product was derived from dried and crushed cow ovaries, and it was taken orally in the form of a vanilla-flavored pill or tablet [1]. Ovarin was sold until the early 1930s, at which time products derived from the urine of pregnant women were developed. Due to limited quantities of estrogens found in human urine and the high cost of their recovery [2], other natural sources were sought. In the 1930s, Bernhard Zondek discovered that the urine of pregnant mares contained large quantities of estrogens [2], and it was from this source that products such as Premarin® (conjugated equine estrogens or CEE) were derived in the late 1930s [1, 2]. Premarin® was eventually approved by the U.S. Food and Drug Administration (FDA) in 1942. Prior to this, Searle introduced the first estrogen patch in 1928 [3], and in 1938, biochemist Charles Dodds published the formula for the synthetic estrogen diethylstilbestrol (DES). The FDA approved DES for the treatment of menopausal symptoms in 1941 [1]. While a number of different products for the treatment of menopausal symptoms were introduced over the ensuing decades, Premarin® remains the leading hormone-based product.

It is by no coincidence that Premarin® is still the dominant hormone-based product for the treatment of menopausal symptoms. Prior to 1962, drugs merely needed to demonstrate safety and not efficacy to gain FDA approval [1]. Therefore, Premarin® was never subjected to today's rigorous FDA approval standards, one of which is that the active ingredient(s) must be clearly defined and characterized. To this day, the active components of Premarin® have still not been completely defined [4]. In 1997, the FDA's Center for Drug Evaluation and Research (CDER) announced that generic forms of Premarin® would no longer be approved. Due to concerns over lack of bioequivalence, safety and efficacy, prior approvals of such products were revoked under a proposal endorsed by the FDA's Generic Drugs Advisory Committee in 1991 [1]. Until the active ingredients of Premarin® have been fully characterized, it will remain difficult if not impossible to prove bioequivalence, which is a requirement for generic drugs. Therefore, as a result of strict FDA rules to which it was never subjected, the manufacturer of Premarin® has a de facto monopoly on the market for conjugated equine estrogens. In our opinion, under today's FDA regulations, it is highly unlikely that Premarin® would even have been approved in the first place.

Based on an assessment performed under a program called the Drug Efficacy Study Implementation (DESI), which is designed to evaluate the efficacy of drugs that had been approved prior to 1962, the FDA announced in 1972 that several different estrogen-based products, including Premarin®, were effective for the treatment of menopausal symptoms [1]. Since the approval of Premarin® in 1942, the use of estrogen-based products as menopausal hormone therapy steadily increased until 1975, when reports of an increased risk of endometrial cancer [5, 6] led to a dramatic reduction. Once the protective effects of progestin on the endometrium became established, and estrogens were considered effective therapy for osteoporosis (i.e. bone loss), the use of estrogen-based menopausal hormone therapy resurged through 2001 [1]. Another contributing factor to the popularity of these products was the belief that estrogen provided a coronary heart disease (CHD) benefit, which was backed by clinical evidence [7-11]. In 2002, results of the Women's Health Initiative (WHI) trial of estrogen plus progestin in postmenopausal women with a uterus showed that hormone replacement therapy (HRT) was associated with increased risks of breast cancer and coronary heart disease, which led to early termination of this trial [12]. As a result of the findings in this trial as well as the WHI's trial of estrogen alone in postmenopausal women without a uterus [13], the use of hormone replacement therapy declined precipitously, and interest was sparked in the development of new non-hormonal compounds like ospemifene (see Chapter 4) for the treatment of menopausal symptoms.

Although the FDA has approved synthetic forms of estrogen for use in the treatment of menopausal symptoms, this Chapter will focus on Premarin® (conjugated equine estrogens), as it is by far the most commonly prescribed form of estrogen for use as hormone replacement therapy. Throughout this Chapter, we will be using the term hormone replacement therapy to refer to either estrogen monotherapy, meaning treatment with estrogen alone, or therapy with an estrogen combined with a progestin when the context applies to either treatment. When the context applies specifically to estrogen or estrogen plus progestin, the appropriate terms will be used.

What, Exactly, Is Premarin®?

Premarin® (conjugated equine estrogens) is prescribed for the treatment of menopausal symptoms, including vasomotor symptoms (i.e. hot flashes and night sweats) and the symptoms of vulvar and vaginal atrophy (VVA), which include vaginal dryness and painful sexual intercourse (dyspareunia). It is a form of hormone replacement therapy intended to increase the level of estrogen in a woman's body once natural production declines as a result of menopause. As mentioned in the Introduction to this Chapter, Premarin® is a product derived from pregnant mares' urine, which contains copious amounts of different estrogens [2]. While eleven different active estrogen compounds have been identified (see Figure 3.1), Premarin® contains numerous other as yet unidentified molecules that are thought to include more estrogens, progestins and even androgens, which are the primary sex hormones in men. In total, Premarin® may contain up to an astounding 230 different molecules [4]. If the known health risks (discussed below) are not enough to complicate a postmenopausal woman's decision regarding the use of Premarin® to treat her menopausal symptoms, the production process of this product adds an element of social conscience that must be considered. Whether administered in tablet or cream form, the active ingredients in Premarin® are derived from pregnant mares' urine (hence the name... PREgnant MARes' urINe). Debate over the handling protocol of female horses for the production of Premarin® has advocates on both sides. Some believe that the value of Premarin® to humans outweighs the consequences to lesser mammals. However, many animal activist groups find the impact on horses to be appalling [14-16].

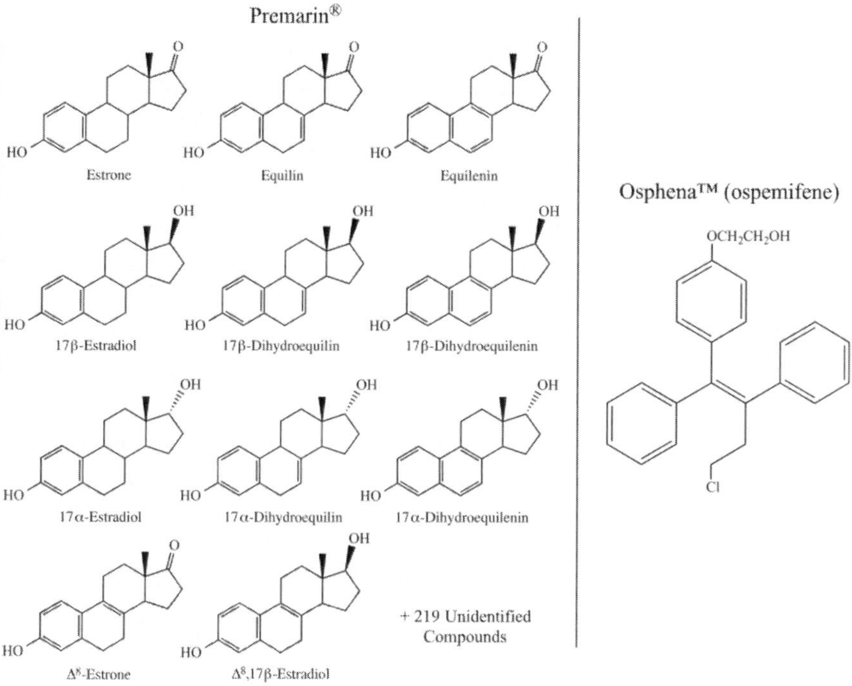

Figure 3.1. Chemical structures of Premarin® and Osphena™ (ospemifene).

Initially, a select group of female horses are intentionally impregnated for the sole purpose of increasing the levels of estrogen in their urine. A horse pregnancy lasts for eleven months, and during that time each mare is restricted to a confinement stall with limited mobility for up to 20 hours a day. While in that stall, a urine collection device is strapped to the horse. The urine of several horses is then combined and processed into either a tablet that can be consumed by a postmenopausal woman, or a cream that can be applied to a woman's skin. Once a horse's pregnancy reaches term, the foal is typically taken away from its mother and transferred to a farm for some other purpose. Meanwhile, the mother is re-impregnated and the process starts all over again for her. The mare lives through up to twelve consecutive pregnancies until she can no longer bear offspring, and then she too is transferred to a farm. There are a number of potential outcomes for the mares and foals from this process, but they are not the topic of this book.

In our opinion, by today's stricter FDA standards for drug approval, Premarin® likely would never have even made it into human clinical trials, let alone mass production. In 1942 when Premarin® was first approved for sale in the United States, the regulatory requirements for FDA approval were arcane relative to today's rigorous criteria. At that time, the FDA was bound only by the Federal Food, Drug, and Cosmetic Act of 1938 that required new drugs to be shown safe before being marketed to the public. Since then, several government acts and amendments have been put in place to more effectively protect the public, including but not limited to specific procedures for the appraisal of the toxicity of chemicals in 1949, the appointment of FDA consumer consultants in 1952, a substantial expansion of FDA staff and facilities in 1955, a consumer bill of rights in 1962, a bioresearch monitoring program in 1977, new regulations for human subjects in 1981, the Food and Drug Administration Modernization Act of 1997, and the formation of the Drug Safety Board in 2005.

While the process for decomposing and hydrolyzing pregnant mares' urine results in effective estrogen concentrations, it also results in concentrations of a variety of many other currently unidentified molecules [4]. The vast majority of these other molecules are largely unknown and untested regarding biologic activity and potential side effects in humans. In addition, each individual horse will carry its own unique set of hormones and by-products based on its body composition, genetics, age, diet, and environmental conditions. Combining the urine of several individual horses produces a cocktail of unknown impact to a postmenopausal woman. Every batch of Premarin® is required to have a consistent concentration of estrogen, but each batch will also have a unique set of additional molecules based on the particular horses that contributed their waste product to its production. The variability alone would likely prohibit Premarin® from being approved by the FDA today, but the toxicities from even a consistent set of known molecules would certainly require a fresh set of studies to ensure that the ingredients in Premarin® do not promote previously unidentified long-term side effects. Today's strict FDA rules have also hamstrung the manufacturer of Premarin® by forcing them to continue to produce this product from the urine of pregnant mares. It may be of value to have a policy change and allow manufacturers to have exclusive rights to use other sources of conjugated estrogens.

What Are the Benefits of Using Premarin® As Hormone Replacement Therapy?

Numerous studies have demonstrated that Premarin® is effective in treating common menopausal maladies including vasomotor symptoms (i.e.

hot flashes and night sweats), the principal symptoms of vulvar and vaginal atrophy (i.e. vaginal dryness and dyspareunia), and in the prevention of osteoporosis (i.e. bone loss). Other more controversial benefits include prevention of coronary heart disease and neurodegenerative disorders such as Alzheimer's disease, the most common form of dementia. The results of the WHI and other clinical studies called these latter benefits into serious question, and the debate over whether hormone replacement therapy offers any protection from coronary heart disease or cognitive decline is still ongoing. To be clear, estrogen-based menopausal hormone therapies, including Premarin®, have neither been approved nor are recommended for the treatment or prevention of coronary heart disease, dementia or any other chronic disease. Current treatment guidelines call for the use of the lowest effective dose for the shortest possible duration consistent with treatment goals [17, 18].

Vasomotor Symptoms

As mentioned in Chapter 1, hot flashes and night sweats, collectively known as vasomotor symptoms (VMS), are the most commonly encountered and problematic symptoms experienced by women as they progress through the menopausal transition, with up to 80% of women experiencing vasomotor symptoms to some degree. While lifestyle modifications such as stopping smoking, limiting alcohol consumption and weight loss tend to make vasomotor symptoms less bothersome, the effect is limited, and thus women experiencing more severe symptoms would likely benefit most from hormone therapy [19]. Premarin®, either with or without a progestin, typically medroxyprogesterone acetate (MPA), which is commonly used in birth control preparations, is the most effective therapy for menopausal vasomotor symptoms and associated problems such as poor sleep quality, difficulty concentrating, and irritability that can lead to an overall reduced quality of life [17, 20, 21]. The primary indication for the use of menopausal hormone therapy is the treatment of moderate to severe vasomotor symptoms, and nearly all of the systemically administered hormone therapy products, with the exception of the ultralow-dose estrogen patch used for the prevention of osteoporosis, are FDA approved for this indication [17]. Estrogen has been shown to reduce both the severity and frequency of vasomotor symptoms by over 75%, typically within a month of starting treatment [22, 23]. For women unable to take products containing estrogen for their vasomotor symptoms due to other health conditions, the commonly used progestin medroxyprogesterone acetate has been shown to be very effective in the management of vasomotor symptoms, although the use of medroxyprogesterone acetate in women with a history of breast cancer is not advised [23-25]. Recently, in 2013, the FDA approved the first non-hormonal treatment for vasomotor symptoms. The drug paroxetine, sold under the trade name Paxil® for the treatment of depression, is from a class of antidepressants known as selective serotonin reuptake inhibitors (SSRIs), and it was found to be effective in reducing the incidence of hot flashes at a low dose of 7.5 mg [19, 26]. For the treatment of moderate to severe hot flashes, low-dose paroxetine is sold under the trade name Brisdelle®.

Vulvar and Vaginal Atrophy (VVA)

Unlike vasomotor symptoms, which tend to resolve over time, the symptoms of vulvar and vaginal atrophy (i.e. vaginal dryness, dyspareunia, itching) are chronic and progressive without treatment. Vulvar and vaginal atrophy is commonly referred to as atrophic vaginitis when inflammation is present. Prior to the approval of ospemifene in 2013 (see Chapter 4), the only effective prescription treatments for vulvar and vaginal atrophy were estrogen-based hormonal therapies. Over-the-counter lubricants and moisturizers are available and recommended for postmenopausal women experiencing mild symptoms, but these remedies are generally ineffective for women suffering from moderate to severe vulvar and vaginal atrophy symptoms, and they do nothing to address the underlying condition [27]. Most of the orally administered estrogen therapy products and all of the local vaginal estrogen products such as Premarin® Vaginal Cream are FDA approved for the treatment of vulvar and vaginal atrophy and its associated symptoms. For women experiencing symptoms of vulvar and vaginal atrophy in the absence of vasomotor symptoms, locally applied estrogen products are recommended as lower doses with less frequent administration have been shown to be effective, and low-dose vaginal estrogens can be used without a progestin in postmenopausal women with a uterus [18].

Vaginal estrogen therapy has actually been shown to be more effective in treating the symptoms of vulvar and vaginal atrophy compared to orally administered preparations [28, 29]. Some systemic absorption does occur with continued use of locally applied therapies, however, and long-term safety data are lacking [18, 30]. Patients should report any unusual bleeding to their doctors as soon as possible so they may be thoroughly evaluated for uterine safety. Locally administered, low-dose vaginal estrogens for the treatment of vulvar and vaginal atrophy are available as creams, tablets and rings.

Osteoporosis

The connection between bone loss after menopause and low ovarian hormone levels was first reported in the *Journal of the American Medical Association* in 1941 by Albright and colleagues [31]. At 50 years of age, a woman's lifetime risk of experiencing a bone fracture due to osteoporosis is approximately 60%, and the specific risk of a hip fracture is 16% [2]. Contributing to this risk is the fact that, early in menopause, there is a 5-7 year period of rapid bone loss during which bone mineral density in the spine may decrease by up to 30%. Bone mineral density is a measure of calcium and other minerals in the bone as a means of estimating bone strength. Following this period, bone loss continues at a much slower rate [23]. Osteoporosis has a significant impact on the overall health of postmenopausal women, and the risk of death is greatly increased following an osteoporotic hip or spinal fracture [32]. To achieve the greatest benefit in those women at high risk of osteoporosis, treatment should be initiated soon after menopause to prevent the rapid loss of bone mass.

In 1972, the FDA announced that Premarin® and other estrogen products were likely effective for osteoporosis prevention [1]. Ten years later, intermediate doses of Premarin® were found to maintain bone mineral density more effectively compared to lower doses of Premarin® or placebo in women who had undergone surgical menopause, or removal of their ovaries [33]. A few years later in 1986, the FDA published another announcement stating that Premarin® was indeed effective for preventing osteoporosis [1], an indication for which Premarin® was later approved. Since then, numerous clinical trials have established that both standard and low-dose estrogen-based hormone therapies are effective in the prevention and treatment (standard doses only) of postmenopausal osteoporosis. A three-year clinical trial, known as the Postmenopausal Estrogen-Progestin Interventions (PEPI) study, clearly showed the benefits of Premarin® in preserving bone mineral density in the spine and hip compared to a placebo [34]. Other studies have shown that standard doses of estrogen-based hormone therapy are effective in reducing bone fractures in the hip, spine and other regions by up to 50% when started soon after menopause, a benefit that was not limited to just women with osteoporosis [35-37]. Even low doses of estrogen therapy were found to significantly increase bone mineral density compared to a placebo [38, 39]. In spite of the reduced osteoporotic bone fracture benefits, neither Premarin® nor any of the other estrogen-based menopausal therapies have been FDA approved for the treatment of osteoporosis. It should also be pointed out that while Premarin® is very effective in preserving bone mineral density and preventing fractures in both healthy postmenopausal women and those with osteoporosis, these benefits disappear rapidly upon discontinuation of treatment [40, 41]. Within just a few years of stopping estrogen therapy in the WHI estrogen-alone trial, the incidence of hip fracture in the placebo-treated and estrogen-treated patients was the same [41]. While long-term use of estrogen therapy is an option for women at high risk of fractures due to osteoporosis—there is no evidence to suggest that long-term therapy is ineffective—the risk of serious side effects increases with the duration of treatment.

What about the Coronary Heart Disease and Cognition Benefits of Premarin®?

Prior to the results of the Heart and Estrogen/progestin Replacement Study (HERS), which studied estrogen plus progestin, and the WHI trials of estrogen plus progestin and estrogen alone, numerous observational studies suggested that Premarin® significantly reduced the risk of coronary heart disease. The results of larger randomized controlled trials, however, have shown that estrogen either alone or in combination with a progestin, does not have such clear benefits. In the case of estrogen and progestin combined therapy, the risk of coronary heart disease was actually increased [12], and while estrogen alone did not increase the risk of coronary heart disease, it provided no overall benefit either [13]. Similarly, with respect to cognitive performance and dementia, there are data suggesting that hormone therapy may have a beneficial effect on cognitive performance and help prevent dementia (Alzheimer's disease) in postmenopausal women [42-44]. However, there are a number of more recent randomized controlled trials showing either no benefit or a detrimental effect on cognitive decline and Alzheimer's disease, especially for estrogen plus progestin [45]. Clearly, the data do not support the use of hormonal therapy to prevent or treat coronary heart disease or cognitive decline, and Premarin® is not indicated for either of these conditions [46]. The clinical data regarding the effects of hormonal therapy on coronary heart disease and cognitive performance and dementia are discussed below.

Premarin® and Coronary Heart Disease

One of the earliest published studies on the effects of hormone replacement therapy on coronary heart disease events was the Framingham Heart Study, which showed that the risk of cardiovascular disease was almost doubled with the use of estrogen over an eight-year period [47]. Appearing in the same issue of the *New England Journal of Medicine* was the Nurses' Health Study, the results of which showed that the risk of coronary heart disease in women who had *ever* used estrogen was approximately half that in women who had *never* used estrogen [11]. Fundamental differences in these two studies such as the inclusion in the Framingham Study of cardiovascular events other than heart attack and coronary heart disease are believed to have accounted for the disagreement in the results [1]. The findings of several later studies agreed with the Nurses' Health Study, showing a reduced risk of coronary heart disease associated with the use of estrogens [8-10]. By 1991, the preponderance of the evidence indicated that the use of Premarin® without a progestin, known as unopposed estrogen therapy, resulted in a significant reduction in the risk of coronary heart disease [7], leading to an FDA Advisory Committee voting to recommend an indication of coronary heart disease risk reduction for unopposed estrogen therapy in postmenopausal women. Interestingly, the FDA, which usually accepts the recommendations of its Advisory Committees, never acted on this recommendation. In 1992, a meta-analysis, which is a combined analysis of the results of multiple studies, was published showing that the use of unopposed estrogen resulted in a one-third reduction in the risk of fatal heart disease. This paper went on to suggest that this benefit would save more lives than those endangered by the combined increased risk of breast and uterine cancers because heart disease is far more prevalent [48]. A later meta-analysis published in 1998, prior to the results of controlled clinical trials, again showed a coronary heart disease risk reduction benefit with the use of unopposed estrogen therapy, which predominated at that time in the United States, and that this benefit was also seen with the use of estrogen plus progestin [49]. This publication did point out, however, that the known biases in the observational studies may be exaggerating the benefits of estrogen, and that in the absence of data from randomized controlled clinical trials, hormone replacement therapy should not be universally recommended for reducing the risk of coronary heart disease [49]. Results from later clinical trials began to reveal that the apparent coronary heart disease benefits of hormone replacement therapy were not what they appeared to be.

The Heart and Estrogen/progestin Replacement Study (HERS) was the first large clinical trial that was designed specifically to assess whether the risk of coronary heart disease events in postmenopausal women with known coronary disease is reduced with the use of estrogen plus progestin therapy [3, 50]. Interestingly, while this study was originally designed to evaluate both unopposed estrogen and estrogen plus progestin therapies, the company funding the trial decided to focus instead on estrogen plus progestin therapy in postmenopausal women with a uterus. It is thought that the company made this modification to the original study design with the expectation that they would receive FDA approval for a statement to the effect that unopposed estrogen is beneficial for the heart [3]. This approval, however, was never issued. The HERS trial included 2,763 postmenopausal women assigned to either placebo or treatment with a tablet containing conjugated equine estrogens and the progestin medroxyprogesterone acetate. After an average of approximately four years of treatment, the results showed that there was no difference in combined nonfatal heart attacks and coronary heart disease-related deaths between the hormone replacement therapy and placebo groups, even though a highly significant decrease in low-density lipoprotein (LDL), the so-called "bad" cholesterol, and an increase in high-density lipoprotein (HDL), the so-called "good" cholesterol, were observed in the women who received hormone replacement therapy compared to placebo. Notably, while no difference was seen overall, hormone replacement therapy was found to significantly increase the risk of coronary heart disease events during the first year of treatment [50]. Although the data suggested a trend in coronary heart disease benefit with continued use beyond the first year, 2-3 years of additional follow-up did not show any evidence of long-term coronary heart disease benefit with hormone replacement therapy [51]. Other than heart attacks and coronary heart disease-related deaths, stroke and peripheral artery disease were also evaluated, and again, no differences were seen between the treatment groups [52, 53]. Given the results of all the previous studies, the outcome of HERS came as a complete surprise. However, a much older study known as the Coronary Drug Project performed in men with established heart disease showed that conjugated equine estrogens increased the incidence of heart attacks and blood clotting (thromboembolic) events [54, 55].

The Heart and Estrogen/progestin Replacement Study was what is known as a secondary prevention trial. That is, it evaluated whether hormone replacement therapy had any benefit in preventing additional coronary heart disease events in women with established coronary heart disease. Following the HERS, the results of several additional secondary prevention trials evaluating conjugated equine estrogens alone, conjugated equine estrogens plus progestin, and non-conjugated equine estrogen regimens were reported. As in the HERS trial, some of these studies reported no overall coronary heart disease benefit [56-59], while some of them actually showed harmful effects of hormone therapy [60, 61]. Although it was not designed to assess the effects of hormonal therapy on disease, the Postmenopausal Estrogen-Progestin Interventions trial mentioned earlier found a higher incidence of cardiovascular and blood clotting events in women taking estrogen plus progestin for three years [34]. Based on all of these trials, it would thus appear that postmenopausal women with established heart disease are already beyond the point where hormonal treatment with either unopposed estrogen or estrogen plus progestin would be of any benefit, and the previously reported coronary heart disease benefits of estrogen therapy in healthy women may not be as clear-cut as once thought. Interest began to build in the WHI trials funded by the National Institutes of Health (NIH), trials that would assess both unopposed estrogen and estrogen plus progestin as primary prevention of coronary heart disease. Primary prevention trials evaluate the effectiveness of a treatment in a healthy population, which in this case would be postmenopausal women with no history of heart disease.

In 1992, the United States Congress solicited a report from the Office of Technology Assessment (OTA) that emphasized the need to conduct clinical trials in order to assess the health effects of menopausal estrogen/progestin therapy. To help address this need, the NIH funded the Women's Health Initiative (WHI) trials of estrogen alone in postmenopausal women without a uterus and estrogen plus progestin in postmenopausal women with a uterus. These trials were specifically designed to address the effects of hormonal therapy compared to a placebo on the incidence of coronary heart disease (nonfatal heart attacks and death due to coronary heart disease) as well as to evaluate the overall risks and benefits of hormonal therapy in predominantly healthy postmenopausal women. The incidence of invasive breast cancer was the primary adverse event measured in these trials [12, 13]. After an average of 5.2 years of treatment, the combined estrogen/progestin trial, which enrolled a total of 16,608 postmenopausal women aged 50-79 years, was stopped early due to an increased risk of breast cancer and the fact that overall risks had exceeded benefits. The initial results showed that the risk of coronary heart disease was significantly increased with hormone treatment compared to placebo, more so in the first year of treatment [12]. Final results from this trial showed that overall coronary heart disease risk was still increased with hormone treatment compared to placebo, but the difference was no longer significant [62]. When the estrogen alone trial, which enrolled a total of 10,739 postmenopausal women aged 50-79 years, showed a significantly increased risk of stroke and failed to demonstrate any clear coronary heart disease benefit or any overall health benefits, the decision was made to terminate this trial early as well after an average of 6.8 years of treatment [13].

The latest follow-up data from the estrogen alone trial still showed no overall coronary heart disease benefits [41, 63]. Interestingly, the risk of coronary heart disease in the patients treated with estrogen/progestin that had been significantly elevated in the initial results had become nearly neutral approximately eight years after stopping treatment [63]. Needless to say, the results of these trials showing no benefit on coronary heart disease with estrogen alone and harmful effects with estrogen plus progestin came as a bit of a shock to the medical community, who had believed that the treatments would show some degree of beneficial effect. As a result of the findings from these clinical trials, there was a sharp decline in the number of prescriptions for Premarin® and Prempro® (conjugated equine estrogens plus medroxyprogesterone acetate) and other orally administered estrogens.

The debate surrounding the coronary heart disease benefits of estrogen continued long after publication of the WHI trials results, with critics pointing to key differences between the observational studies and the WHI trials. Perhaps the biggest difference was that the average age of the women participating in the WHI trials was 63, while many of the women in the observational studies of coronary heart disease risk were under the age of 55 when they began their hormone therapy [17]. As it turns out, this difference may be important. When data from the WHI estrogen/progestin trial was reanalyzed based on time since menopause when the women began treatment, the risk of coronary heart disease was slightly reduced compared to placebo in those women who were less than 10 years past menopause when they started treatment, a population more representative of the women actually being treated with hormonal therapy. The risk of coronary heart disease tended to increase with time since menopause [64]. Reanalysis of data from the estrogen alone WHI trial based on age and time since menopause showed that coronary heart disease risk was reduced, similar to the older observational studies, in younger, more recently menopausal women [64, 65], an effect that was more pronounced when reassessed four years after treatment ended [41]. When data from both of the WHI trials was combined, there was a tendency for women starting hormone therapy less than 10 years from menopause to have a *reduced* coronary heart disease risk, and women starting therapy more than 10 years after menopause to have an *increased* risk [64]. However, when data from both of these trials was combined with data from the WHI observational study, the risk of coronary heart disease did not vary based on when hormone therapy was initiated [66]. The WHI observational study included a total of 93,676 postmenopausal women who were ineligible or unwilling to participate in the WHI clinical trials of estrogen alone and estrogen plus progestin, and it was intended to provide information on risk factors for major causes of disease and death in postmenopausal women [67]. Finally, a study involving 1,006 healthy postmenopausal women aged 45-58 showed that after approximately 10 years of hormonal therapy—synthetic estrogen alone in hysterectomized women and synthetic estrogen plus a progestin in women with a uterus—and an additional six years of follow-up, women treated with hormonal therapy had a significantly reduced risk of death, heart failure and heart attacks [68].

Lower doses of estrogen have also been investigated with respect to the risk of coronary heart disease in postmenopausal women. While long-term safety data on low-dose hormonal therapy with estrogen or estrogen/progestin is limited, the data that is available suggest that the risk of coronary heart disease in younger, more recently menopausal women is not adversely affected [69]. In a study involving 4,065 postmenopausal women with an average age of 53 years, 1,662 of whom received low-dose conjugated equine estrogens alone or in combination with medroxyprogesterone acetate, there were no cases of heart attack or death due to cardiovascular disease observed [70]. In the Nurses' Health Study, the risk of coronary heart disease in those women receiving lower doses of estrogen was reduced, although the number of women taking lower doses in this trial was limited [71]. A recently completed clinical trial known as the Kronos Early Estrogen Prevention Study (KEEPS), which assessed the effects of oral, low-dose conjugated equine estrogens and transdermal estrogen compared to placebo on cognition and coronary heart disease in recently postmenopausal women, was designed to address the shortcomings of previous clinical trials, including the WHI [72]. Unfortunately, the results of this trial have not yet been published.

Based on all of this clinical data, the benefits of hormone replacement therapy in coronary heart disease still remain unclear, and if there is any benefit at all, it appears to be confined to those women who begin unopposed estrogen-based hormonal therapy soon after menopause, but the benefits even in this setting remain controversial. In the absence of definitive clinical data showing clear benefits, hormone replacement therapy cannot be recommended for the prevention or treatment of heart disease in postmenopausal women of any age.

Premarin®, Cognitive Performance and Dementia

As in the case of the coronary heart disease benefits of estrogen, early studies pointed to the potential benefits of hormone therapy with respect to cognitive performance and dementia, the most common form of which is Alzheimer's disease [42-44]. However, the evidence supporting a beneficial effect of estrogen on cognition and dementia in postmenopausal women remains quite limited. The Study of Women's health Across the Nation (SWAN) (see Chapter 1) found that the menopausal transition does appear to have a small but significant effect on cognitive performance, but this effect does not appear to be permanent [73] and cannot be accounted for by menopausal symptoms [74]. The SWAN study showed a beneficial cognitive effect of hormonal therapy in women who initiated treatment prior to their final menstrual period and then stopped, while women who started treatment after their final menstrual period experienced a detrimental effect [73]. The Nurses' Health Study, which has been following over 100,000 female nurses since 1976, showed that long-term use of hormonal therapy in postmenopausal women who began treatment shortly after menopause had no benefit on cognitive function, and it may in fact have accelerated a decline in cognitive performance [75]. Another study in 1,889 postmenopausal women with an average age of 74.5 years, called the Cache County Study, found that previous or current use of hormonal therapy exceeding 10 years reduced the risk of Alzheimer's disease [44, 76]. Two randomized controlled clinical trials of conjugated equine estrogens in women with established Alzheimer's disease found that hormonal therapy produced no benefits [77, 78].

The largest clinical trial evaluating the effects of hormonal therapy on cognitive performance and dementia conducted to date is the Women's Health Initiative Memory Study (WHIMS), an ancillary study to the WHI clinical trials discussed earlier. Like the WHI trials, WHIMS had two components: a study in which women received daily estrogen plus progestin (0.625 mg conjugated equine estrogens + 2.5 mg medroxyprogesterone acetate) and a study in which women were given 0.625 mg conjugated equine estrogens alone daily. The estrogen/progestin study enrolled a total of 4,532 postmenopausal women aged 65-79 years and free of dementia. When global cognitive function was assessed in the estrogen/progestin study after an average of just over four years of treatment, the women treated with hormonal therapy had a significant decline in their cognitive performance score compared to the women treated with placebo [45]. Even more troubling was that the risk of dementia was doubled with hormone treatment, which resulted in 19 more cases of dementia compared to placebo. Alzheimer's disease was the most common form of dementia observed. This risk translates to an additional 23 cases of dementia per 10,000 women per year, a difference that was found to be statistically significant. When mild cognitive impairment was considered, no meaningful differences were observed between the groups [79]. In the estrogen-alone study, which enrolled a total of 2,947 postmenopausal women aged 65-79 years and free of dementia, treatment with conjugated equine estrogens for an average of 5.4 years was found to significantly decrease cognitive performance [80]. As in the estrogen plus progestin trial, the incidence of dementia was also increased by 12 cases per 10,000 women per year with hormone treatment compared to placebo, but this difference was not significant. While no meaningful difference in the incidence of mild cognitive impairment was seen with estrogen treatment compared to placebo, when the incidences of dementia and mild cognitive impairment were combined, a significant increase was observed with estrogen treatment [81]. When the data from both arms of the WHIMS trial were combined, a highly significant decrease in overall cognitive performance and highly significant increases in the incidence of dementia and mild cognitive impairment were observed [80, 81]. When global cognitive performance was reassessed approximately seven years after treatment ended, no meaningful differences in cognitive function were seen regardless of the type of hormone therapy in younger postmenopausal women aged 50-55 years at the start of treatment [82]. It has been hypothesized that the increased risk of thrombosis, or blood clotting, in older postmenopausal women may at least partially account for the increased risk of cognitive decline and dementia seen with hormonal therapy in these women [46, 83].

Given the conflicting data surrounding the effects of postmenopausal hormone therapy with estrogen alone or estrogen combined with a progestin on cognition and dementia, and the potential for harmful effects found in the Women's Health Initiative Memory Study, the use of estrogen-based hormonal therapy with or without a progestin for the prevention or treatment of these or any other chronic conditions associated with menopause is currently neither recommended nor approved by the FDA.

What Are the Known Side Effects of Premarin®?

Unfortunately, the known side effects of Premarin® force many postmenopausal women to make a tough decision between getting relief for their menopausal symptoms and placing themselves at risk for side effects. The clinically proven benefits of reducing hot flashes, night sweats and vaginal discomfort, along with the potential to slow the development of osteoporosis, must be weighed against the increased risks of blood clots, strokes, endometrial cancer, breast cancer, heart disease and dementia [46]. As mentioned earlier, it was the increased risk of breast cancer that resulted in early termination of the WHI study of estrogen plus progestin, and the increased risk of stroke combined with no clear coronary heart disease benefits that led to the early stoppage of the WHI estrogen-alone trial [12, 13]. Thirty years prior to this in 1973, a clinical trial of Premarin® for the prevention of heart attacks and strokes was abruptly halted when it was discovered that the patients, men with known heart disease, actually experienced an increase in blood clots and heart attacks [54, 55]. Then in 1975, the *New England Journal of Medicine* published two articles showing evidence that endometrial cancer risk increased with the use of estrogen replacement therapy [5, 6]. A meta-analysis performed 20 years later confirmed a significantly increased risk of endometrial cancer with the use of unopposed estrogen [84]. The FDA mandated labeling changes for estrogen products the following year highlighting the increased risk of uterine cancer from long-term use of estrogens [1]. It was later established that the addition of a progestin to hormone therapy could protect the endometrium from the potentially carcinogenic effects of estrogen, and estrogen plus progestin hormone replacement therapy became standard treatment in postmenopausal women with an intact uterus [1]. In the WHI estrogen plus progestin trial, following 13 years of cumulative follow-up, the risk of endometrial cancer in women receiving hormonal therapy was actually significantly reduced compared to the women given placebo [63].

New research over the years has continued to reveal additional risks. More than a decade after the elevated risk of endometrial cancer was revealed, a 1989 study found an increased risk of breast cancer with estrogen replacement therapy [85]. The increased risk of breast cancer was later confirmed in the WHI trial of estrogen plus progestin, which found an increased risk of invasive breast cancer following approximately five years of treatment [12]. Eight years later, the risk of invasive breast cancer was still significantly higher in the women who had received estrogen/progestin treatment [63]. Interestingly, the risk of invasive breast cancer has remained consistently lower in the women who received estrogen in the WHI estrogen-alone trial [13, 41, 63]. In 1997, the FDA announced that generic versions of Premarin® would no longer be approved, citing the need to protect the public (see Introduction to this Chapter). Then in 2002, as previously discussed, government scientists terminated the Women's Health Initiative study of estrogen plus progestin, stating clear evidence that long-term use of hormonal therapy significantly increases the risk of breast cancer, strokes, and heart attacks [12]. The following year, the FDA required Premarin® and other estrogen and estrogen/progestin products to carry new warning labels that highlight increased risks of heart disease, stroke, breast cancer, pulmonary embolisms, and blood clots [86]. A pulmonary embolism is a blood clot that becomes lodged in the pulmonary artery, which delivers blood from the heart to the lungs, and it is very dangerous. In 2004, the WHI study of estrogen alone was also stopped earlier than planned due to an increased risk of stroke in the absence of any clear coronary heart disease benefits [13]. An increased risk of ischemic stroke, or stroke caused by clotted blood, has consistently been found in studies of estrogen alone or estrogen combined with a progestin when taken orally [83, 87, 88]. The use of transdermal estrogen may reduce this risk [89, 90]. In 2007, a meta-analysis of primarily observational studies was published that found an increased risk of ovarian cancer associated with the use of hormone replacement therapy [91], a result supported by later research [92]. The WHI trial of estrogen plus progestin found no evidence of an increased risk of ovarian cancer [93]. Two years earlier in 2005, the International Agency for Research on Cancer (IARC), which is the World Health Organization's (WHO) cancer research agency, classified hormone replacement therapy as carcinogenic in humans [94].

More recently, with respect to the increased risk of breast cancer, extended follow-up of the WHI estrogen plus progestin study in 2008 showed that hormone replacement therapy interferes with the detection of breast cancer, leading to late diagnosis of advanced cancer and resulting in a poorer likelihood of survival, an effect that persisted after discontinuation of hormonal therapy [95]. Years later in 2012, data from the earlier mentioned Nurses' Health Study covering a 28-year follow-up period (1980-2008) revealed that long-term use of postmenopausal hormone therapy for 10-15 years increased the risk of developing invasive breast cancer between 22% (estrogen alone) and 88% (estrogen plus progestin). The risk of breast cancer in this study continued to rise with longer use [96].

In 2013, the FDA rejected the new drug applications for two new non-estrogen therapies for menopausal symptoms (Serada™ and LDMP) that would have competed with Premarin®, citing that the overall risk/benefit profiles were not acceptable. The active ingredients in these experimental medications, gabapentin in Serada™ and paroxetine in LDMP, are already FDA approved for the treatment of epilepsy and depression, respectively, and each of these new products was designed to release low doses of their active ingredients. Later in 2013, low-dose paroxetine, currently being sold under the trade name Brisdelle®, was approved for the treatment of hot flashes. For a more comprehensive discussion of the side effects and warnings associated with Premarin®, please refer to Chapter 5: Understanding Side Effects: Boxed Warnings and Package Inserts.

Conclusion

Premarin® (conjugated equine estrogens) is the most commonly prescribed treatment for menopausal symptoms. A product derived from the urine of pregnant mares, Premarin® contains an estimated 230 different compounds, only 11 of which, all estrogens, have been identified. In spite of this, Premarin® has FDA approval because it was never subjected to today's rigorous FDA requirements, many of which were not in place in 1942 when it was originally approved. Premarin® has proven benefits in treating common menopausal maladies such as vasomotor symptoms (i.e. hot flashes and night sweats), the major symptoms of vulvar and vaginal atrophy (i.e. vaginal dryness and dyspareunia), and in preventing postmenopausal osteoporosis. At one time it was widely believed that Premarin® also had benefits in preventing coronary heart disease, cognitive decline and dementia, but numerous studies have failed to demonstrate any clear benefits, with some suggesting harmful effects. The use of Premarin® and other estrogen products for the treatment of postmenopausal women changed dramatically when the results of the Women's Health Initiative studies were announced. These studies showed that Premarin® combined with progestin increased the risk of breast cancer and coronary heart disease, and that Premarin® with or without a progestin increased the risks of stroke and blood clots. The WHI Memory Study additionally showed that Premarin® may be harmful for cognitive function and increases the risk for dementia.

As a result of the WHI trials, Premarin® now carries numerous warnings as discussed in Chapter 5, which deals with understanding the side effects of Premarin® and Osphena™ (ospemifene). As discussed in Chapter 4, ospemifene, a new non-estrogen approved for the treatment of dyspareunia as a result of vulvar and vaginal atrophy due to menopause, is from a family of molecules known as selective estrogen receptor modulators (SERMs), which act like estrogen in some tissues and antiestrogens in other tissues. Other FDA approved SERMs include toremifene, tamoxifen, and raloxifene. Interestingly, the FDA has elected to label ospemifene as if it were an estrogen like Premarin®, but the available data clearly show that this labeling is unwarranted. Ospemifene is a single, well characterized synthetic compound, while Premarin® is composed of numerous different estrogen compounds along with over 200 other unidentified compounds about which the biologic activity and possible side effects can only be speculated (see Figure 3.1). As a SERM, ospemifene should be labeled in a manner consistent with other SERMs like toremifene, of which it is a metabolite, or raloxifene, to which research has shown ospemifene to be the most similar. This issue is discussed in greater detail in Chapter 5.

Recently, in October 2013, the FDA approved a new treatment for menopausal symptoms and the prevention of postmenopausal osteoporosis. This new drug, sold under the trade name Duavee™, is a combination of conjugated estrogens and the SERM bazedoxifene. In clinical studies, this combination was also evaluated as a potential treatment for vulvar and vaginal atrophy using two different formulations (0.45 mg or 0.625 mg conjugated estrogens combined with 20 mg bazedoxifene). When bazedoxifene was combined with the higher dose of conjugated estrogens, significant improvement in vulvar and vaginal atrophy symptoms was seen compared to a placebo, while the combination containing the lower dose of conjugated estrogens proved inferior. This result suggests that the vulvar and vaginal atrophy benefits of this new treatment are derived from the estrogen component rather than bazedoxifene, and thus Duavee™, which failed to receive FDA approval for the treatment of vulvar and vaginal atrophy, cannot be considered a competitor in the same class as ospemifene, which is a non-hormonal agent, due to its reliance on estrogen to achieve its vulvar and vaginal atrophy benefits. The next Chapter discusses the history, development and approval of ospemifene.

References

[1]   Stefanick, M. L. (2005). Estrogens and progestins: background and history, trends in use, and guidelines and regimens approved by the US Food and Drug Administration. *Am J Med, 118 Suppl 12B*, 64-73.

[2]   Davis, S. R., Dinatale, I., Rivera-Woll, L., Davison, S. (2005). Postmenopausal hormone therapy: from monkey glands to transdermal patches. *J Endocrinol, 185(2)*, 207-222.

[3]   Barrett-Connor, E. (2003). Clinical review 162: cardiovascular endocrinology 3: an epidemiologist looks at hormones and heart disease in women. *J Clin Endocrinol Metab, 88(9)*, 4031-4042.

[4]   Bhavnani, B. R., Stanczyk, F. Z. (2014). Pharmacology of conjugated equine estrogens: efficacy, safety and mechanism of action. *J Steroid Biochem Mol Biol, 142*, 16-29.

[5]   Smith, D. C., Prentice, R., Thompson, D. J., Herrmann, W. L. (1975). Association of exogenous estrogen and endometrial carcinoma. *N Engl J Med, 293(23)*, 1164-1167.

[6]   Ziel, H. K., Finkle, W. D. (1975). Increased risk of endometrial carcinoma among users of conjugated estrogens. *N Engl J Med, 293(23)*, 1167-1170.

[7]   Barrett-Connor, E., Bush, T. L. (1991). Estrogen and coronary heart disease in women. *JAMA, 265(14)*, 1861-1867.

[8]   Bush, T. L., Barrett-Connor, E., Cowan, L. D., Criqui, M. H., Wallace, R. B., Suchindran, C. M., et al. (1987). Cardiovascular mortality and noncontraceptive use of estrogen in women: results from the Lipid Research Clinics Program Follow-up Study. *Circulation, 75(6)*, 1102-1109.

[9]   Henderson, B. E., Paganini-Hill, A., Ross, R. K. (1988). Estrogen replacement therapy and protection from acute myocardial infarction. *Am J Obstet Gynecol, 159(2)*, 312-317.

[10]   Petitti, D. B., Perlman, J. A., Sidney, S. (1987). Noncontraceptive estrogens and mortality: long-term follow-up of women in the Walnut Creek Study. *Obstet Gynecol, 70(3 Pt 1)*, 289-293.

[11]   Stampfer, M. J., Willett, W. C., Colditz, G. A., Rosner, B., Speizer, F. E., Hennekens, C. H. (1985). A prospective study of postmenopausal estrogen therapy and coronary heart disease. *N Engl J Med, 313(17)*, 1044-1049.

[12]   Rossouw, J. E., Anderson, G. L., Prentice, R. L., LaCroix, A. Z., Kooperberg, C., Stefanick, M. L., et al. (2002). Risks and benefits of estrogen plus progestin in healthy postmenopausal women: principal results From the Women's Health Initiative randomized controlled trial. *JAMA, 288(3)*, 321-333.

[13]   Anderson, G. L., Limacher, M., Assaf, A. R., Bassford, T., Beresford, S. A., Black, H., et al. (2004). Effects of conjugated equine estrogen in postmenopausal women with hysterectomy: the Women's Health Initiative randomized controlled trial. *JAMA, 291(14)*, 1701-1712.

[14]   Equine-Voices-Rescue-&-Sanctuary. Premarin. Equine Voices Rescue & Sanctuary; 2014 [June 26, 2014]; Available from http://www.equinevoices.org/horses/issues/premarin/.

[15] Mullins, A. One More Reason to Say "No" to Premarin. PETA; 2010 [June 26, 2014]; Available from: http://prime.peta.org.

[16] The-Horse-Fund. Premarin Horses. The Horse Fund; 2014 [June 26, 2014]; Available from: http://www.horsefund.org.

[17] NAMS (2012). The 2012 hormone therapy position statement of: The North American Menopause Society. *Menopause, 19(3)*, 257-271.

[18] NAMS (2013). Management of symptomatic vulvovaginal atrophy: 2013 position statement of The North American Menopause Society. *Menopause, 20(9)*, 888-902.

[19] Al-Safi, Z. A., Santoro, N. (2014). Menopausal hormone therapy and menopausal symptoms. *Fertil Steril, 101(4)*, 905-915.

[20] Barnabei, V. M., Cochrane, B. B., Aragaki, A. K., Nygaard, I., Williams, R. S., McGovern, P. G., et al. (2005). Menopausal symptoms and treatment-related effects of estrogen and progestin in the Women's Health Initiative. *Obstet Gynecol, 105(5 Pt 1)*, 1063-1073.

[21] NIH (2005). National Institutes of Health State-of-the-Science Conference statement: management of menopause-related symptoms. *Ann Intern Med, 142(12 Pt 1)*, 1003-1013.

[22] Nelson, H. D., Haney, E., Humphrey, L., Miller, J., Nedrow, A., Nicolaidis, C., et al. (2005). Management of menopause-related symptoms. *Evid Rep Technol Assess (Summ), (120)*, 1-6.

[23] Shifren, J. L., Schiff, I. (2010). Role of hormone therapy in the management of menopause. *Obstet Gynecol, 115(4)*, 839-855.

[24] Goodwin, J. W., Green, S. J., Moinpour, C. M., Bearden, J. D., 3rd, Giguere, J. K., Jiang, C. S., et al. (2008). Phase III randomized placebo-controlled trial of two doses of megestrol acetate as treatment for menopausal symptoms in women with breast cancer: Southwest Oncology Group Study 9626. *J Clin Oncol, 26(10)*, 1650-1656.

[25] Schiff, I., Tulchinsky, D., Cramer, D., Ryan, K. J. (1980). Oral medroxyprogesterone in the treatment of postmenopausal symptoms. *JAMA, 244(13)*, 1443-1445.

[26] Stearns, V., Slack, R., Greep, N., Henry-Tilman, R., Osborne, M., Bunnell, C., et al. (2005). Paroxetine is an effective treatment for hot flashes: results from a prospective randomized clinical trial. *J Clin Oncol, 23(28)*, 6919-6930.

[27] Burich, R., DeGregorio, M. (2011). Current treatment options for vulvovaginal atrophy. *Expert Rev Obstet Gynecol, 6(2)*, 141-151.

[28] Cardozo, L., Bachmann, G., McClish, D., Fonda, D., Birgerson, L. (1998). Meta-analysis of estrogen therapy in the management of

urogenital atrophy in postmenopausal women: second report of the Hormones and Urogenital Therapy Committee. *Obstet Gynecol, 92(4 Pt 2)*, 722-727.

[29] Long, C. Y., Liu, C. M., Hsu, S. C., Wu, C. H., Wang, C. L., Tsai, E. M. (2006). A randomized comparative study of the effects of oral and topical estrogen therapy on the vaginal vascularization and sexual function in hysterectomized postmenopausal women. *Menopause, 13(5)*, 737-743.

[30] Sturdee, D. W., Panay, N. (2010). Recommendations for the management of postmenopausal vaginal atrophy. *Climacteric, 13(6)*, 509-522.

[31] Albright, F., Smith, P. H., Richardson, A. M. (1941). Postmenopausal osteoporosis: its clinical features. *JAMA, 116(22)*, 2465-2474.

[32] Sanders, S., Geraci, S. A. (2013). Osteoporosis in postmenopausal women: considerations in prevention and treatment: (women's health series). *South Med J, 106(12)*, 698-706.

[33] Genant, H. K., Cann, C. E., Ettinger, B., Gordan, G. S. (1982). Quantitative computed tomography of vertebral spongiosa: a sensitive method for detecting early bone loss after oophorectomy. *Ann Intern Med, 97(5)*, 699-705.

[34] Bush, T. L., Wells, H. B., James, M. K., Barrett-Connor, E., Marcus, R., Greendale, G., et al. (1996). Effects of hormone therapy on bone mineral density: results from the postmenopausal estrogen/progestin interventions (PEPI) trial. The Writing Group for the PEPI. *JAMA, 276(17)*, 1389-1396.

[35] Cauley, J. A., Robbins, J., Chen, Z., Cummings, S. R., Jackson, R. D., LaCroix, A. Z., et al. (2003). Effects of estrogen plus progestin on risk of fracture and bone mineral density: the Women's Health Initiative randomized trial. *JAMA, 290(13)*, 1729-1738.

[36] Cauley, J. A., Zmuda, J. M., Ensrud, K. E., Bauer, D. C., Ettinger, B. (2001). Timing of estrogen replacement therapy for optimal osteoporosis prevention. *J Clin Endocrinol Metab, 86(12)*, 5700-5705.

[37] Jackson, R. D., LaCroix, A. Z., Gass, M., Wallace, R. B., Robbins, J., Lewis, C. E., et al. (2006). Calcium plus vitamin D supplementation and the risk of fractures. *N Engl J Med, 354(7)*, 669-683.

[38] Ettinger, B., Ensrud, K. E., Wallace, R., Johnson, K. C., Cummings, S. R., Yankov, V., et al. (2004). Effects of ultralow-dose transdermal estradiol on bone mineral density: a randomized clinical trial. *Obstet Gynecol, 104(3)*, 443-451.

[39] Prestwood, K. M., Kenny, A. M., Kleppinger, A., Kulldorff, M. (2003). Ultralow-dose micronized 17beta-estradiol and bone density and bone metabolism in older women: a randomized controlled trial. *JAMA, 290(8)*, 1042-1048.

[40] Heiss, G., Wallace, R., Anderson, G. L., Aragaki, A., Beresford, S. A., Brzyski, R., et al. (2008). Health risks and benefits 3 years after stopping randomized treatment with estrogen and progestin. *JAMA, 299(9)*, 1036-1045.

[41] LaCroix, A. Z., Chlebowski, R. T., Manson, J. E., Aragaki, A. K., Johnson, K. C., Martin, L., et al. (2011). Health outcomes after stopping conjugated equine estrogens among postmenopausal women with prior hysterectomy: a randomized controlled trial. *JAMA, 305(13)*, 1305-1314.

[42] Barrett-Connor, E., Laughlin, G. A. (2009). Endogenous and exogenous estrogen, cognitive function, and dementia in postmenopausal women: evidence from epidemiologic studies and clinical trials. *Semin Reprod Med, 27(3)*, 275-282.

[43] Hogervorst, E., Bandelow, S. (2010). Sex steroids to maintain cognitive function in women after the menopause: a meta-analyses of treatment trials. *Maturitas, 66(1)*, 56-71.

[44] Shao, H., Breitner, J. C., Whitmer, R. A., Wang, J., Hayden, K., Wengreen, H., et al. (2012). Hormone therapy and Alzheimer disease dementia: new findings from the Cache County Study. *Neurology, 79(18)*, 1846-1852.

[45] Rapp, S. R., Espeland, M. A., Shumaker, S. A., Henderson, V. W., Brunner, R. L., Manson, J. E., et al. (2003). Effect of estrogen plus progestin on global cognitive function in postmenopausal women: the Women's Health Initiative Memory Study: a randomized controlled trial. *JAMA, 289(20)*, 2663-2672.

[46] Rozenberg, S., Vandromme, J., Antoine, C. (2013). Postmenopausal hormone therapy: risks and benefits. *Nat Rev Endocrinol, 9(4)*, 216-227.

[47] Wilson, P. W., Garrison, R. J., Castelli, W. P. (1985). Postmenopausal estrogen use, cigarette smoking, and cardiovascular morbidity in women over 50. The Framingham Study. *N Engl J Med, 313(17)*, 1038-1043.

[48] Grady, D., Rubin, S. M., Petitti, D. B., Fox, C. S., Black, D., Ettinger, B., et al. (1992). Hormone therapy to prevent disease and prolong life in postmenopausal women. *Ann Intern Med, 117(12)*, 1016-1037.

[49] Barrett-Connor, E., Grady, D. (1998). Hormone replacement therapy, heart disease, and other considerations. *Annu Rev Public Health, 19*, 55-72.

[50] Hulley, S., Grady, D., Bush, T., Furberg, C., Herrington, D., Riggs, B., et al. (1998). Randomized trial of estrogen plus progestin for secondary prevention of coronary heart disease in postmenopausal women. Heart and Estrogen/progestin Replacement Study (HERS) Research Group. *JAMA, 280(7)*, 605-613.

[51] Grady, D., Herrington, D., Bittner, V., Blumenthal, R., Davidson, M., Hlatky, M., et al. (2002). Cardiovascular disease outcomes during 6.8 years of hormone therapy: Heart and Estrogen/progestin Replacement Study follow-up (HERS II). *JAMA, 288(1)*, 49-57.

[52] Hsia, J., Simon, J. A., Lin, F., Applegate, W. B., Vogt, M. T., Hunninghake, D., et al. (2000). Peripheral arterial disease in randomized trial of estrogen with progestin in women with coronary heart disease: the Heart and Estrogen/Progestin Replacement Study. *Circulation, 102(18)*, 2228-2232.

[53] Simon, J. A., Hsia, J., Cauley, J. A., Richards, C., Harris, F., Fong, J., et al. (2001). Postmenopausal hormone therapy and risk of stroke: The Heart and Estrogen-progestin Replacement Study (HERS). *Circulation, 103(5)*, 638-642.

[54] (1970). The Coronary Drug Project. Initial findings leading to modifications of its research protocol. *JAMA, 214(7)*, 1303-1313.

[55] (1973). The Coronary Drug Project. Findings leading to discontinuation of the 2.5-mg day estrogen group. The coronary Drug Project Research Group. *JAMA, 226(6)*, 652-657.

[56] Angerer, P., Stork, S., Kothny, W., Schmitt, P., von Schacky, C. (2001). Effect of oral postmenopausal hormone replacement on progression of atherosclerosis : a randomized, controlled trial. *Arterioscler Thromb Vasc Biol, 21(2)*, 262-268.

[57] Byington, R. P., Furberg, C. D., Herrington, D. M., Herd, J. A., Hunninghake, D., Lowery, M., et al. (2002). Effect of estrogen plus progestin on progression of carotid atherosclerosis in postmenopausal women with heart disease: HERS B-mode substudy. *Arterioscler Thromb Vasc Biol, 22(10)*, 1692-1697.

[58] Cherry, N., Gilmour, K., Hannaford, P., Heagerty, A., Khan, M. A., Kitchener, H., et al. (2002). Oestrogen therapy for prevention of reinfarction in postmenopausal women: a randomised placebo controlled trial. *Lancet, 360(9350)*, 2001-2008.

[59] Herrington, D. M., Reboussin, D. M., Brosnihan, K. B., Sharp, P. C., Shumaker, S. A., Snyder, T. E., et al. (2000). Effects of estrogen

replacement on the progression of coronary-artery atherosclerosis. *N Engl J Med*, *343(8)*, 522-529.

[60] Clarke, S. C., Kelleher, J., Lloyd-Jones, H., Slack, M., Schofiel, P. M. (2002). A study of hormone replacement therapy in postmenopausal women with ischaemic heart disease: the Papworth HRT atherosclerosis study. *BJOG*, *109(9)*, 1056-1062.

[61] Waters, D. D., Alderman, E. L., Hsia, J., Howard, B. V., Cobb, F. R., Rogers, W. J., et al. (2002). Effects of hormone replacement therapy and antioxidant vitamin supplements on coronary atherosclerosis in postmenopausal women: a randomized controlled trial. *JAMA*, *288(19)*, 2432-2440.

[62] Manson, J. E., Hsia, J., Johnson, K. C., Rossouw, J. E., Assaf, A. R., Lasser, N. L., et al. (2003). Estrogen plus progestin and the risk of coronary heart disease. *N Engl J Med*, *349(6)*, 523-534.

[63] Manson, J. E., Chlebowski, R. T., Stefanick, M. L., Aragaki, A. K., Rossouw, J. E., Prentice, R. L., et al. (2013). Menopausal hormone therapy and health outcomes during the intervention and extended poststopping phases of the Women's Health Initiative randomized trials. *JAMA*, *310(13)*, 1353-1368.

[64] Rossouw, J. E., Prentice, R. L., Manson, J. E., Wu, L., Barad, D., Barnabei, V. M., et al. (2007). Postmenopausal hormone therapy and risk of cardiovascular disease by age and years since menopause. *JAMA*, *297(13)*, 1465-1477.

[65] Hsia, J., Langer, R. D., Manson, J. E., Kuller, L., Johnson, K. C., Hendrix, S. L., et al. (2006). Conjugated equine estrogens and coronary heart disease: the Women's Health Initiative. *Arch Intern Med*, *166(3)*, 357-365.

[66] Prentice, R. L., Manson, J. E., Langer, R. D., Anderson, G. L., Pettinger, M., Jackson, R. D., et al. (2009). Benefits and risks of postmenopausal hormone therapy when it is initiated soon after menopause. *Am J Epidemiol*, *170(1)*, 12-23.

[67] Prentice, R. L., Chlebowski, R. T., Stefanick, M. L., Manson, J. E., Langer, R. D., Pettinger, M., et al. (2008). Conjugated equine estrogens and breast cancer risk in the Women's Health Initiative clinical trial and observational study. *Am J Epidemiol*, *167(12)*, 1407-1415.

[68] Schierbeck, L. L., Rejnmark, L., Tofteng, C. L., Stilgren, L., Eiken, P., Mosekilde, L., et al. (2012). Effect of hormone replacement therapy on cardiovascular events in recently postmenopausal women: randomised trial. *BMJ*, *345*, e6409.

[69] Warren, M. P. (2007). Historical perspectives in postmenopausal hormone therapy: defining the right dose and duration. *Mayo Clin Proc*, *82(2)*, 219-226.

[70] Lobo, R. A. (2004). Evaluation of cardiovascular event rates with hormone therapy in healthy, early postmenopausal women: results from 2 large clinical trials. *Arch Intern Med*, *164(5)*, 482-484.

[71] Grodstein, F., Manson, J. E., Stampfer, M. J. (2006). Hormone therapy and coronary heart disease: the role of time since menopause and age at hormone initiation. *J Womens Health (Larchmt)*, *15(1)*, 35-44.

[72] Wharton, W., Gleason, C. E., Miller, V. M., Asthana, S. (2013). Rationale and design of the Kronos Early Estrogen Prevention Study (KEEPS) and the KEEPS Cognitive and Affective sub study (KEEPS Cog). *Brain Res*, *1514*, 12-17.

[73] Greendale, G. A., Huang, M. H., Wight, R. G., Seeman, T., Luetters, C., Avis, N. E., et al. (2009). Effects of the menopause transition and hormone use on cognitive performance in midlife women. *Neurology*, *72(21)*, 1850-1857.

[74] Greendale, G. A., Wight, R. G., Huang, M. H., Avis, N., Gold, E. B., Joffe, H., et al. (2010). Menopause-associated symptoms and cognitive performance: results from the study of women's health across the nation. *Am J Epidemiol*, *171(11)*, 1214-1224.

[75] Kang, J. H., Weuve, J., Grodstein, F. (2004). Postmenopausal hormone therapy and risk of cognitive decline in community-dwelling aging women. *Neurology*, *63(1)*, 101-107.

[76] Zandi, P. P., Carlson, M. C., Plassman, B. L., Welsh-Bohmer, K. A., Mayer, L. S., Steffens, D. C., et al. (2002). Hormone replacement therapy and incidence of Alzheimer disease in older women: the Cache County Study. *JAMA*, *288(17)*, 2123-2129.

[77] Mulnard, R. A., Cotman, C. W., Kawas, C., van Dyck, C. H., Sano, M., Doody, R., et al. (2000). Estrogen replacement therapy for treatment of mild to moderate Alzheimer disease: a randomized controlled trial. Alzheimer's Disease Cooperative Study. *JAMA*, *283(8)*, 1007-1015.

[78] Wang, P. N., Liao, S. Q., Liu, R. S., Liu, C. Y., Chao, H. T., Lu, S. R., et al. (2000). Effects of estrogen on cognition, mood, and cerebral blood flow in AD: a controlled study. *Neurology*, *54(11)*, 2061-2066.

[79] Shumaker, S. A., Legault, C., Rapp, S. R., Thal, L., Wallace, R. B., Ockene, J. K., et al. (2003). Estrogen plus progestin and the incidence of dementia and mild cognitive impairment in postmenopausal women: the

Women's Health Initiative Memory Study: a randomized controlled trial. *JAMA, 289(20)*, 2651-2662.

[80] Espeland, M. A., Rapp, S. R., Shumaker, S. A., Brunner, R., Manson, J. E., Sherwin, B. B., et al. (2004). Conjugated equine estrogens and global cognitive function in postmenopausal women: Women's Health Initiative Memory Study. *JAMA, 291(24)*, 2959-2968.

[81] Shumaker, S. A., Legault, C., Kuller, L., Rapp, S. R., Thal, L., Lane, D. S., et al. (2004). Conjugated equine estrogens and incidence of probable dementia and mild cognitive impairment in postmenopausal women: Women's Health Initiative Memory Study. *JAMA, 291(24)*, 2947-2958.

[82] Espeland, M. A., Shumaker, S. A., Leng, I., Manson, J. E., Brown, C. M., LeBlanc, E. S., et al. (2013). Long-term effects on cognitive function of postmenopausal hormone therapy prescribed to women aged 50 to 55 years. *JAMA Intern Med, 173(15)*, 1429-1436.

[83] Lobo, R. A., Clarkson, T. B. (2011). Different mechanisms for benefit and risk of coronary heart disease and stroke in early postmenopausal women: a hypothetical explanation. *Menopause, 18(2)*, 237-240.

[84] Grady, D., Gebretsadik, T., Kerlikowske, K., Ernster, V., Petitti, D. (1995). Hormone replacement therapy and endometrial cancer risk: a meta-analysis. *Obstet Gynecol, 85(2)*, 304-313.

[85] Bergkvist, L., Adami, H. O., Persson, I., Hoover, R., Schairer, C. (1989). The risk of breast cancer after estrogen and estrogen-progestin replacement. *N Engl J Med, 321(5)*, 293-297.

[86] US-Food-and-Drug-Administration. Estrogen and Estrogen with Progestin Therapies for Postmenopausal Women. FDA; 2010 [July 11, 2014]; Available from: http://www.fda.gov/Drugs/ DrugSafety/InformationbyDrugClass/ucm135318.htm.

[87] Bath, P. M., Gray, L. J. (2005). Association between hormone replacement therapy and subsequent stroke: a meta-analysis. *BMJ, 330(7487)*, 342.

[88] Sare, G. M., Gray, L. J., Bath, P. M. (2008). Association between hormone replacement therapy and subsequent arterial and venous vascular events: a meta-analysis. *Eur Heart J, 29(16)*, 2031-2041.

[89] Renoux, C., Dell'aniello, S., Garbe, E., Suissa, S. (2008). Hormone replacement therapy use and the risk of stroke. *Maturitas, 61(4)*, 305-309.

[90] Sweetland, S., Beral, V., Balkwill, A., Liu, B., Benson, V. S., Canonico, M., et al. (2012). Venous thromboembolism risk in relation to use of

different types of postmenopausal hormone therapy in a large prospective study. *J Thromb Haemost, 10(11)*, 2277-2286.

[91] Greiser, C. M., Greiser, E. M., Doren, M. (2007). Menopausal hormone therapy and risk of ovarian cancer: systematic review and meta-analysis. *Hum Reprod Update, 13(5)*, 453-463.

[92] Pearce, C. L., Chung, K., Pike, M. C., Wu, A. H. (2009). Increased ovarian cancer risk associated with menopausal estrogen therapy is reduced by adding a progestin. *Cancer, 115(3)*, 531-539.

[93] Anderson, G. L., Judd, H. L., Kaunitz, A. M., Barad, D. H., Beresford, S. A., Pettinger, M., et al. (2003). Effects of estrogen plus progestin on gynecologic cancers and associated diagnostic procedures: the Women's Health Initiative randomized trial. *JAMA, 290(13)*, 1739-1748.

[94] Mueck, A. O., Seeger, H. (2008). The World Health Organization defines hormone replacement therapy as carcinogenic: is this plausible? *Gynecol Endocrinol, 24(3)*, 129-132.

[95] Chlebowski, R. T., Anderson, G., Pettinger, M., Lane, D., Langer, R. D., Gilligan, M. A., et al. (2008). Estrogen plus progestin and breast cancer detection by means of mammography and breast biopsy. *Arch Intern Med, 168(4)*, 370-377; quiz 345.

[96] Chen, W. Y., Willett, W. C., Hankinson, S. E., Rosner, B. A., editors. Long-term use of hormone thrapy and breast cancer incidence and mortality (Abstract LB-60). American Association of Cancer Research Annual Meeting; March 31-April 4, 2012; Chicago, IL: AACR.

Chapter 4

Osphena™ (Ospemifene): History, Development and FDA Approval of a Non-estrogen

Abstract

After over 20 years in development, Osphena™ (ospemifene) was approved by the U.S. Food and Drug Administration (FDA) in February 2013 for the treatment of moderate to severe dyspareunia (i.e. painful sexual intercourse) associated with vulvar and vaginal atrophy (VVA) due to menopause. As the first non-hormonal, non-estrogen treatment for this indication available in the United States, the approval of ospemifene represents a significant milestone in postmenopausal women's health. Due to the potentially serious side effects associated with hormone replacement therapy (HRT), as discussed in Chapter 3, that have come to light since the announcement of the results of the Women's Health Initiative Studies of estrogen plus progestin and estrogen alone in postmenopausal women in 2002 and 2004, respectively, the use of estrogen-based hormonal therapies for the treatment of menopausal symptoms has been declining, creating an unmet medical need for safe and effective, non-estrogen alternatives. With the approval of ospemifene, for the first time doctors now have an effective, non-estrogen option to conventional hormonal therapies, which contain estrogen, commonly in the form of conjugated equine estrogens (CEE), for the treatment of vulvar and vaginal atrophy. Ospemifene is in a class of drugs known as selective estrogen receptor modulators (SERMs), a class which includes a number of other drugs such as tamoxifen and toremifene, which are used in breast cancer treatment and prevention (tamoxifen only), and raloxifene, which is used in the treatment and prevention of osteoporosis as well as breast cancer prevention. Similar to these other compounds, ospemifene possesses a unique mix of estrogenic and antiestrogenic tissue-specific effects in bone, breast and vagina, and because of these effects, ospemifene is also referred to as an estrogen receptor agonist/antagonist. Among the different SERMs that have been approved for clinical use, ospemifene is unique in that it exerts a nearly full estrogen agonist effect in the vagina, while having neutral to slight estrogenic effects in the lining of the uterus, or endometrium. These qualities make ospemifene well suited for the treatment of dyspareunia associated with vulvar and vaginal atrophy, which affects up to 60% of postmenopausal women. This Chapter discusses the history, preclinical and clinical development, known and potential side effects and the FDA approval of ospemifene.

Introduction

Ospemifene is an estrogen receptor agonist/antagonist, also known as a selective estrogen receptor modulator (SERM), a drug class that includes tamoxifen and toremifene, which are used in the treatment and prevention (tamoxifen only) of breast cancer, and raloxifene, which is used in the treatment and prevention of osteoporosis as well as the prevention of breast cancer. These drugs are called SERMs because of the way in which they interact with the estrogen receptors found in different tissues. In some tissues like bone, they act like estrogen (agonist effect), and in other tissues like the breast, they act as antiestrogens (antagonist effect). Each of these drugs has a unique profile of estrogen agonist and antagonist effects. For example, tamoxifen is antiestrogenic in breast tissue, which makes it an effective breast cancer treatment, but in the lining of the uterus, or endometrium, tamoxifen stimulates the tissue like estrogen, which can lead to the development of uterine cancer [1]. However, raloxifene, which is also antiestrogenic in the breast, has no significant agonist effects in the uterus [2, 3]. Unwanted estrogenic effects in the uterus have proven to be a major impediment to the development of new SERM-like drugs, with several experimental compounds having been dropped from clinical development due to this side effect [4]. Tamoxifen was actually the first clinically useful SERM, and when it was recognized that tamoxifen was having mixed estrogenic and antiestrogenic effects in different tissues, the search began for newer compounds that have desirable estrogenic effects in tissues like bone, while avoiding potentially serious estrogenic effects in tissues like the uterus. Raloxifene was originally developed as a breast cancer treatment, but it failed in clinical trials [5]. Data demonstrating positive effects of raloxifene on bone mineral density [2], a property it shares with the other SERMs, led to its successful development for the prevention and treatment of osteoporosis, indications for which it received U.S. Food and Drug Administration (FDA) approval in 1997 and 1999, respectively. Raloxifene was additionally approved for the prevention of invasive breast cancer in 2007 following the results of the Study of Tamoxifen and Raloxifene [6]. Ospemifene is a direct result of the search for a new estrogen agonist/antagonist with beneficial effects on bone and serum cholesterol, neutral to antagonistic effects in the uterus, and antiestrogenic effects in the breast. Among the different SERMs that have been FDA approved, ospemifene is unique because it has a nearly full estrogen agonist effect in the vagina, making it an effective treatment for vulvar and vaginal atrophy (VVA) [7-10], while tamoxifen may aggravate this condition [11].

After nearly 22 years in development, ospemifene, sold under the trade name Osphena,™ was approved by the FDA in February 2013 for the treatment of moderate to severe dyspareunia associated with vulvar and vaginal atrophy due to menopause [12]. Ospemifene is the first non-hormonal, non-estrogen treatment approved for this use and represents a significant milestone in postmenopausal women's health. Prior to the approval of ospemifene, the only other approved treatments for this condition contained estrogen, which when taken orally had been associated with an increased risk of breast cancer [13] and other potentially serious complications [14-16] in large clinical trials of hormone replacement therapy. There was thus an unmet medical need for an effective, non-estrogen treatment for the symptoms of vulvar and vaginal atrophy. Uniquely among the FDA-approved SERMs, which include tamoxifen, toremifene, raloxifene, clomiphene and bazedoxifene (when combined with conjugated estrogens), ospemifene exerts a strong, beneficial estrogen agonist effect on the vaginal epithelium, a property that was first observed in Phase I clinical trials [17]. In clinical drug development, Phase I is the earliest phase where experimental drugs are evaluated for safety as well as how they are metabolized and excreted. The recognition of ospemifene's strong estrogenic effects in the vagina ultimately led to its development as a treatment for dyspareunia rather than postmenopausal osteoporosis and breast cancer prevention, which were the originally targeted indications.

This Chapter will discuss the preclinical and clinical development history of ospemifene from its discovery through FDA approval, its proposed mechanism of action, and its tissue-specific effects on bone, breast, serum cholesterol and vagina. The Chapter will conclude with a discussion of the potential application of ospemifene for the chemoprevention of breast cancer, where a number of preclinical studies in rats and mice have shown ospemifene to be as effective as tamoxifen, and the controversy surrounding the FDA's questionable decision to label ospemifene as if it were an estrogen rather than a SERM.

Preclinical Development

1. How Was Ospemifene Discovered and What Was the Focus of Early Preclinical Development?

Ospemifene was selected from a group of related chemical compounds called triphenylethylenes in the early 1990s for study as a potential treatment for postmenopausal osteoporosis, or bone loss. As discussed in Chapter 1, osteoporosis occurs when the rate of bone resorption (i.e. the breaking down of bone) is no longer balanced with the rate of bone formation, which can occur in postmenopausal women as a result of low circulating levels of estrogen. The combined activities of bone resorption and bone formation are referred to as bone turnover or bone remodeling. The result of this imbalance is a net loss of bone mineral density and weak, porous bone that is at a greatly increased risk of fracture, especially in the wrists, spine, and hip. Ospemifene was selected for study on the basis of what was known about the activity of related compounds in bone. It was known at the time that some metabolites of tamoxifen, which is chemically related to ospemifene, were estrogenic while others were antiestrogenic [18, 19]. A metabolite is a metabolic breakdown product of a drug. When a drug is consumed, enzymes in the liver chemically alter it so that the body can more easily eliminate it either through the urine or feces. Some drugs, known as prodrugs, actually require metabolic conversion to their active forms in order to produce the desired effects. Ospemifene is in the metabolic pathway of the breast cancer drug toremifene, which is also chemically related to tamoxifen. The chemical structure of ospemifene is shown in Figure 3.1 (Chapter 3).

At the time of its discovery, it was reasoned that ospemifene may be useful in the regulation of bone remodeling [20, 21] and that it may have applications in other estrogen-responsive tissues such as the vagina. It was further reasoned that ospemifene could potentially be used as an alternative to hormone replacement therapy. The initial preclinical research was directed towards developing ospemifene for the treatment and prevention of osteoporosis in postmenopausal women. Also studied were the effects of ospemifene on serum cholesterol and its genotoxic potential, or its ability to alter DNA, which is a way of assessing a drug's potential to cause cancer. When a drug or one of its metabolites binds to DNA, the result is what is known as a DNA adduct. The formation of DNA adducts has been associated with the development of cancer. For example, it is well known that tamoxifen has been associated with the development of endometrial cancer, and the formation of DNA adducts may be involved [22]. Later research then focused on the use of ospemifene in breast cancer chemoprevention as well as the treatment of vulvar and vaginal atrophy, for which ospemifene appeared to be well-suited based on the results of early clinical trials.

2. What Is Ospemifene's Mechanism of Action?

As a SERM, ospemifene primarily acts by binding to estrogen receptors, although the way in which drugs like ospemifene act on a tissue-selective basis is still not completely understood. Two types of estrogen receptors, known as alpha and beta, have so far been identified. The estrogen receptor is part of a superfamily of related receptors that includes the androgen, vitamin D and progesterone receptors. When ospemifene binds to the estrogen receptor, the receptor then translocates into the nucleus of the cell where the DNA is found. The receptor then latches on to particular sequences of DNA that are specific for the estrogen receptor, where it can then affect the expression of certain genes that contain these sequences. When the estrogen receptor is bound to an agonist like estrogen, gene expression is activated, and when it is bound to an antagonist, gene expression is deactivated. Unlike estrogen, which always acts as an agonist, ospemifene can act as either an agonist or antagonist depending on the tissue. It is thought that the basis for this selective action is related to the availability of certain regulatory proteins and the specific conformational change of the receptor after binding ospemifene [23-25]. Like other SERMs, ospemifene changes the three-dimensional shape of the receptor after binding, which, depending on the availability of certain stimulatory and inhibitory cofactors, can result in either agonistic or antagonistic activity [26-28].

3. What Is the Carcinogenic Potential of Ospemifene?

The carcinogenic potential of ospemifene, or its ability to cause cancer, was evaluated in mice, rats, and rhesus macaque monkeys by measuring DNA adducts as discussed above. Using two different strains of laboratory mice, ospemifene was compared to tamoxifen and toremifene with respect to the formation of liver DNA adducts in three different studies [29]. In separate experiments, the drugs were administered both orally and by subcutaneous injection (i.e. injection under the skin) and at standard as well as high doses. Regardless of the dose level, type of mouse, or route of administration, liver DNA adducts were observed only in those mice treated with tamoxifen, and the number of adducts increased with dose [29]. These results were in agreement with another study showing that a major metabolite of tamoxifen more readily reacted with DNA to form adducts compared to the analogous toremifene metabolite [30] and with a study in rats where DNA adducts were seen only in the animals treated with tamoxifen compared to those treated with ospemifene [31]. Toremifene is closely related to tamoxifen, differing by a single chlorine atom that is thought to interfere with how the drug reacts with DNA, potentially preventing the formation of DNA adducts and, subsequently, cancer [22, 29, 30]. Ospemifene, which is in the metabolic pathway of toremifene, may also benefit from this reduced genotoxic, or carcinogenic potential.

Finally, the formation of DNA adducts in the liver and endometrium was assessed in rhesus macaque monkeys following 12 weeks of daily ospemifene dosing. No evidence of DNA adducts was observed either before, during or after treatment. To make sure the DNA adduct test was working, rhesus macaque DNA in test tubes was reacted with a tamoxifen metabolite known to cause DNA adducts and with ospemifene. Adducts were only detected in the DNA reacted with the tamoxifen metabolite [32]. Taken together, the results of all of these studies suggest that ospemifene has a low carcinogenic potential, which is critical now that otherwise healthy women are taking ospemifene to treat dyspareunia associated with vulvar and vaginal atrophy due to menopause.

4. What Are the Effects of Ospemifene in the Bone?

Early in its development, ospemifene was first studied for its effects on bone. In mouse bone marrow cells grown in culture, ospemifene, similar to estrogen, induced the development of osteoblasts (i.e. bone building cells) [33]. In human osteoclasts (i.e. bone resorbing cells) grown in culture, ospemifene and tamoxifen inhibited cell development and bone resorption, effects that were dependent on the presence of the estrogen receptor. Interestingly, tamoxifen's effects were direct while ospemifene required the presence of osteoblasts (i.e. bone building cells) to mediate its effects [34]. In human bone cancer cells derived from osteoblasts and that had been artificially implanted with both types of estrogen receptor (alpha and beta), ospemifene, similar to estrogen, was able to prevent chemotherapy-induced cell death while tamoxifen offered no protection. In the same cells, both ospemifene and estrogen prevented the production of chemical messengers that increase the activity of osteoclasts (i.e. bone resorbing cells), but they acted through different mechanisms [35]. The results of these early studies showed that ospemifene and tamoxifen are estrogen-like in their effects on bone, that is to say beneficial, but their mechanisms differ, which is in keeping with the unique tissue-selective properties of these interesting compounds.

Additional bone experiments were performed in female rats that had their ovaries removed, which has proven to be a good animal model of postmenopausal osteoporosis. Surgical removal of the ovaries is commonly referred to as ovariectomy or oophorectomy. In one study, groups of rats were treated with a control solution, a low dose of ospemifene or a high dose of ospemifene daily for four weeks. Rats given the control solution experienced significant bone loss, while those treated with ospemifene at the higher dose showed significant preservation of bone volume and strength in the femur and spine. The higher dose of ospemifene also significantly reduced measures of bone turnover, which encompasses both bone resorption and the production of new bone, compared to the control animals. When ospemifene and estrogen were combined, no meaningful differences were observed compared to estrogen alone, which indicates that ospemifene did not oppose the effects of estrogen [31]. In another four-week rat study comparing ospemifene to raloxifene, which is a SERM approved for the treatment and prevention of postmenopausal osteoporosis, ospemifene prevented increases in urinary indicators of bone turnover similar to raloxifene [31]. Ospemifene also significantly reduced the number of bone resorbing cells (i.e. osteoclasts), an effect that increased with dose, while raloxifene had no demonstrable effect [36].

In order to determine whether ospemifene's bone-sparing effects are maintained in the long term, female ovariectomized rats (i.e. rats that had their ovaries removed) were treated with ospemifene daily for a full year. The results showed that, similar to the four-week studies, ospemifene significantly prevented losses in bone mineral density and strength compared to untreated control animals [36]. Thus, ospemifene's bone-sparing effects were maintained long-term, which is important for any potential clinical application of ospemifene for the treatment or prevention of postmenopausal osteoporosis. Overall, the results of these early bone studies showed that ospemifene is effective in preventing bone loss in the rat model of postmenopausal osteoporosis, similar to raloxifene, and thus ospemifene should be tested in clinical trials for the treatment and/or prevention of osteoporosis in postmenopausal women. In Phase II clinical trials, discussed later in this Chapter, the effects of ospemifene on key urinary indicators of bone turnover compared to placebo and to raloxifene were explored.

5. What Are the Effects of Ospemifene in the Breast?

The effects of ospemifene in normal breast tissue and breast cancer have been extensively evaluated in tissue culture-based studies and in rat and mouse models of breast cancer. Like all of the other FDA-approved SERMs that have been mentioned—tamoxifen, toremifene and raloxifene—ospemifene has been shown to act as an antiestrogen in breast tissue in both cell culture dish studies and animal studies. This section will first discuss research done in cell culture-based studies of both normal breast tissue and breast cancer, followed by a discussion of all of the animal-based studies evaluating the potential of ospemifene as a breast cancer treatment and preventive agent.

Using well-known human breast cancer cells that express the estrogen receptor and require estrogen for growth, a group of researchers found that ospemifene had no substantial effect on cell growth at concentrations ranging from very low to very high [31]. Another group reported that ospemifene produced a moderate, dose-dependent growth inhibitory effect at a similar range of concentrations, meaning that the inhibitory effect increased as the dose increased. This latter group also studied the effects of ospemifene's main metabolite, a compound called 4-hydroxyospemifene, and found that it produced a stronger growth inhibitory effect than ospemifene in these breast cancer cells, but curiously the inhibitory effect of this compound was apparently unrelated to the dose [37]. When the latter research group repeated these studies using human breast cancer cells that neither express the estrogen receptor nor require estrogen for growth, the growth inhibitory effects of ospemifene and its metabolite were not seen, which suggests that expression of the estrogen receptor is required in order for ospemifene to exert its growth inhibitory effects in breast cancer [37]. In support of this observation, both ospemifene and its metabolite were found to inhibit the expression of a known estrogen-regulated gene in human breast cancer cells at the same drug concentrations [37], a result also reported by the former research group [31]. More recently, when ospemifene and its metabolite were combined with estrogen, they antagonized the expression of an estrogen-regulated gene in human breast cancer cells [38].

In normal human mammary tissue grown in culture dishes, ospemifene was found to exert antiestrogenic, growth inhibitory effects that were similar to raloxifene and tamoxifen [39]. The mammary gland tissue was exposed to ospemifene, raloxifene or tamoxifen at low to moderate concentrations for up to 14 days. Cellular proliferation was assessed after seven days in culture, and ospemifene, similar to tamoxifen and raloxifene, was found to inhibit cell growth in a dose-dependent fashion. This inhibitory effect persisted after 14 days at all doses of ospemifene tested, but interestingly not for the lower doses of tamoxifen and raloxifene [39]. Given the complex mechanisms through which these drugs exert their effects, this result was not unexpected.

The effects of ospemifene on normal breast tissue were also studied in three experiments utilizing rats [40]. As in the normal human mammary tissue study discussed above, ospemifene was found to exert a largely antiestrogenic effect on cellular proliferation and tissue morphology. In these studies, the rats were treated with ospemifene, tamoxifen, raloxifene or estrogen daily for up to 28 days. The proliferation of breast tissue was found to be significantly lower in all three studies following treatment with ospemifene, tamoxifen and raloxifene compared to the rats treated with estrogen or a related synthetic compound called ethinyl estradiol, both of which had a very strong stimulatory effect. When the morphology of the mammary gland was examined, no meaningful induction of mammary gland lobes was observed in the SERM-treated rats. In fact, the number of lobe-like structures was significantly lower in these rats compared to the control rats, which still had intact ovaries [40]. In rats treated with ospemifene or raloxifene, levels of prolactin, a hormone that induces the production of milk, were significantly lower compared to the rats treated with estrogen [40]. To summarize, in breast cancer cell cultures, normal human breast tissue cultures, and normal rat mammary tissue, ospemifene was shown to have antiestrogenic effects that were similar to tamoxifen and raloxifene, both of which have been approved for the prevention of breast cancer in women at high risk.

To evaluate the potential of ospemifene as a breast cancer treatment and chemopreventive agent, several different studies were performed using mouse and rat models of breast cancer. The first two studies were conducted using nude mice without ovaries that had been implanted with human breast tumor tissue dependent on estrogen for growth [31, 37]. Nude mice are a special strain of hairless research mice that have compromised immune systems, rendering them unable to reject foreign tissue. In these studies, human breast cancer cells were injected into the mice to form tumors. The first of these two studies allowed tumors to develop over an eight-week period, after which the mice were treated with ospemifene daily for 48 days [31]. During the eight-week tumor growth period, each mouse had an estrogen pellet implanted beneath the skin that slowly released estrogen to support tumor growth. As pointed out earlier, these particular human breast cancer cells require estrogen for growth. The pellets were removed just prior to ospemifene treatment. The results showed that ospemifene not only failed to support tumor growth, but that tumor volumes decreased in all of the ospemifene-treated mice [31]. In the second study, mice began treatment with ospemifene seven days prior to implantation of breast cancer cells, with treatment continuing daily throughout the study. At all dose levels tested, ospemifene significantly inhibited tumor growth compared to control mice. When this study was repeated using human breast cancer cells that do not depend on estrogen for growth and do not express estrogen receptor alpha, ospemifene had no apparent effect on tumor growth [37]. These two studies showed that not only does ospemifene lack estrogenic activity in breast tumors, but it also acts as an antiestrogen in an estrogen receptor-dependent fashion, results that are consistent with earlier studies. Two recent publications describe these studies and the breast cancer studies that follow in greater detail [41, 42].

The effects of ospemifene in breast cancer were further explored in chemically-induced rat and mouse models, a model in which precancerous breast tissue is transplanted into the mammary glands of host mice, and a model in which breast cancer develops spontaneously under the influence of a gene that had been artificially inserted into the mouse's DNA. In the chemically-induced rat breast cancer model, a chemical carcinogen was given to the animals to cause breast cancer to develop. The breast tumors were allowed to grow for eight weeks before starting ospemifene treatment, which was given daily for four weeks. Tumor growth was then monitored for six weeks following cessation of ospemifene dosing. Except for the lowest dose of ospemifene, the number of breast tumors per rat was significantly lower in all ospemifene-treated groups compared to the control rats that received no ospemifene treatment. When breast tumors were assessed on the basis of whether they were growing, stationary, or regressing, ospemifene was found to reduce the number of growing tumors and increase the number of stationary and regressing tumors in response to dose compared to the control animals. At the highest dose of ospemifene tested, the number of breast tumors was reduced by nearly two-thirds compared to the number of tumors in the control rats [31]. In this rat study, ospemifene was used in a treatment capacity, and the results were consistent with previous studies showing that ospemifene is antiestrogenic in breast tissue.

Two additional studies utilizing the same chemical carcinogen were performed in mice to evaluate the potential of ospemifene to prevent breast cancer [43]. Compared to rats, where only a single dose of the chemical is needed, mice require multiple doses over time to cause breast cancer. Mice in these studies were also implanted with time-release steroid pellets to enhance the formation of breast tumors. The first of these studies compared ospemifene to tamoxifen and raloxifene, all of which were given daily for 37 weeks. Both ospemifene and tamoxifen significantly prevented the formation of breast tumors compared to untreated control mice, with tumor incidence rates of 6% and 0%, respectively. Raloxifene failed to demonstrate any significant antitumor effects in this study [43]. The second study compared ospemifene to tamoxifen over a longer, 52-week period. Both drugs were administered daily throughout the study. As observed in the first study, ospemifene had a highly significant breast cancer preventive effect, with only 5% of mice developing breast cancer compared to none in the tamoxifen-treated mice [43]. These two studies demonstrated that ospemifene may be an effective breast cancer chemopreventive agent, with an efficacy similar to tamoxifen.

The potential of ospemifene as a breast cancer chemopreventive agent was further explored in a unique mouse model in which precancerous breast tissue is transplanted into the mammary glands of genetically similar host mice, thus preventing tissue rejection. The way in which breast cancer develops from the implanted tissue in this model very closely resembles human breast carcinogenesis (i.e. the process of cancer development), making it a good model to study potential treatment and preventive agents [44]. Starting seven days prior to transplantation of precancerous breast tissue and continuing for up to 10 weeks thereafter, groups of mice were treated daily with ospemifene, tamoxifen or control solution. At three weeks post-transplantation, treatment with ospemifene and tamoxifen resulted in significantly smaller precancerous growths compared to control mice [45]. At 10 weeks after transplantation, the incidence of breast tumors as well as the overall size of the implanted tissue was significantly lower in the ospemifene- and tamoxifen-treated mice compared to the untreated control mice. Both ospemifene and tamoxifen significantly inhibited cellular proliferation. When the precancerous tissue was evaluated for the expression of estrogen receptor alpha, ospemifene was found to have significantly increased expression while tamoxifen significantly decreased expression, suggesting that ospemifene and tamoxifen were working through different mechanisms [45]. While interesting from a scientific point of view, such a finding is again not surprising given the complex nature of these medications. The results of this study reinforced the potential of ospemifene as an effective breast cancer chemopreventive agent, similar to tamoxifen.

Most recently, ospemifene was evaluated in both a breast cancer preventive and treatment capacity [46] using an immunologically intact mouse model in which breast cancer develops spontaneously under the influence of a gene that causes breast tissue to rapidly transform into precancerous tissue, with the eventual development of breast cancer in all 10 of the mouse's mammary glands [47]. This model is related to the transplant model discussed above in that these mice are the source of the precancerous transplant tissue. In the prevention study, mice were treated daily with ospemifene at three different doses for 21 weeks. Early in the study, average tumor volumes decreased in response to dose, with the decrease becoming significant at the highest ospemifene dose level. Overall survival, which increased in response to dose and was the main endpoint of this study, was significantly longer in mice receiving the highest dose of ospemifene [46]. Similar results were seen in the breast cancer treatment study, where breast tumors were allowed to develop for 16 weeks prior to treatment with ospemifene. Overall survival was again significantly increased at the highest dose of ospemifene [46]. The results of these two studies showed that ospemifene acts as an antiestrogen in both a treatment and preventive capacity in a mouse model of spontaneous breast cancer that closely resembles human breast carcinogenesis.

6. What Are the Effects of Ospemifene on the Uterus and Endometrium?

As mentioned in the Introduction, adverse estrogenic effects in the uterus have proven to be a major stumbling block in the development of new SERMs [48]. The effects of ospemifene in the uterus and endometrium, which is the inner lining of the uterus, have been extensively evaluated in preclinical animal models, including rats and rhesus macaque monkeys. Clinical effects of ospemifene in these tissues will be discussed later in this Chapter. The rat model of menopause is commonly used to assess the estrogenic effects of drugs in the uterus. Groups of rats that had their ovaries removed were treated daily for four weeks with different doses of ospemifene ranging from low to high or a fixed dose of raloxifene, which is considered to be neutral to antagonistic in the uterus. At the higher doses of ospemifene, uterine weight was significantly increased similar to raloxifene [31]. The highest dose of ospemifene had a slight estrogenic effect on the endometrium; however, none of the ospemifene-treated rats exhibited any evidence of increased cell growth, known as hyperplasia, while 90% of the estrogen-treated control rats showed severe hyperplasia. When administered together, ospemifene antagonized the activity of estrogen. Similarly, in immature rats treated with very low to very high doses of ospemifene, relative uterine weight increased in response to dose, but when combined with estrogen, ospemifene again displayed antagonistic activity. In contrast, when female adult rats that still had their ovaries were treated daily with ospemifene for four weeks, decreases in uterine weight were observed [31]. When higher doses of ospemifene were given to rats without ovaries daily for two weeks, a slight but significant increase in uterine weight was seen, which was again comparable to raloxifene. These increases were, however, still less than half of those seen in response to treatment with estrogen [38]. A single-dose study performed in rats without ovaries compared ospemifene, raloxifene and tamoxifen to estradiol and showed that ospemifene and raloxifene did not significantly increase uterine weight [49]. Finally, in a 52-week study where rats without ovaries were treated with ospemifene daily at three different dose levels, uterine weight was significantly increased at all doses compared to control rats without ovaries, but these increases were still only about half of those seen in the control rats that still had their ovaries [36].

The effects of ospemifene on the uterus and endometrium have also been studied in female rhesus macaque monkeys [32]. Six normally cycling female monkeys ranging in age from 9 to 17 years were treated once a week with ospemifene for three weeks. These animals were examined sonographically 1-3 days prior to treatment, during treatment, and then 4-5 days following their final dose. Assessments of uterine size, shape, contour, position and texture, as well as the appearance of the uterine cavity and endometrial thickness were included in the evaluations. Consistent with the results seen in clinical trials as discussed below, no significant changes in uterine volume or endometrial thickness were observed at any point during treatment [32].

7. What Are the Effects of Ospemifene in the Vagina?

The effects of ospemifene on vaginal weight and epithelial height were examined in three studies utilizing the rat model of menopause [38, 39]. The vaginal epithelium is the outermost layer of tissue lining the vagina, and it is highly responsive to estrogen and estrogen-like compounds. In the first study, groups of rats were treated with three different doses of ospemifene daily for 2-4 weeks and compared to rats treated with raloxifene, estrogen or control (no treatment). When compared to the control rats, all three doses of ospemifene at both two and four weeks of treatment resulted in significantly increased vaginal weight and epithelial height that did not significantly differ from rats treated with estrogen, which was suggestive of a full estrogen agonist effect [38]. In contrast, raloxifene produced increases in vaginal weight and epithelial height only one-half and one-tenth that of estrogen, respectively. This result was expected because raloxifene has not been shown to have any meaningful effects on the vaginal epithelium [39].

Utilizing the same rat model of menopause, the effects of both ospemifene and its metabolite 4-hydroxyospemifene on vaginal weight and epithelial height were evaluated and compared to the hormone ethinyl estradiol, which is a synthetic estrogen, in two additional experiments [38]. A derivative of estradiol, which is the major form of estrogen found in the body, ethinyl estradiol is commonly used in oral birth control preparations. Different groups of rats were given a range of doses from very low to high for ospemifene and its metabolite daily for two weeks compared to a fixed dose of ethinyl estradiol. Both ospemifene and its metabolite were very effective in increasing epithelial height, with a clear dose-response effect observed for ospemifene. All doses of ospemifene tested except for the lowest dose produced a significant increase in epithelial height, while the three highest doses significantly increased vaginal weight compared to the control rats. For ospemifene's metabolite, only the highest dose significantly increased vaginal weight. Ospemifene's maximal effect on epithelial height was approximately equal to that of ethinyl estradiol, suggesting a full estrogen agonist effect, while the effect of the 4-hydroxyospemifene metabolite was suggestive of a partial estrogen agonist effect. When vaginal tissues were examined microscopically, ospemifene treatment resulted in increased thickness and mucification of the epithelium [38]. Mucification is the formation of cells that produce mucus, which provides the natural lubrication of the vagina.

Two studies were performed to specifically evaluate the effects of ospemifene on vaginal tissues in the rat model of menopause [38]. The first of these was a pilot study in which ospemifene was given orally or by vaginal suppository daily for 14 days and compared to orally administered ethinyl estradiol. Ospemifene, whether given orally or by suppository increased the thickness of the vaginal epithelium and increased the expression of progesterone receptor in the epithelium as well as the underlying elastic and muscular tissue layers in a manner similar to ethinyl estradiol. The progesterone receptor is encoded by a gene regulated by estrogen, and thus increased expression of this receptor is an indication of estrogenic activity. To confirm the results of the pilot study, a second study with the same design was conducted examining the effects of ospemifene compared to ethinyl estradiol on the vaginal epithelium and the expression of the progesterone receptor. Again, regardless of the route of drug administration, orally or locally, the effects of ospemifene on the thickness of the vaginal epithelium and expression of the progesterone receptor in the epithelium and underlying tissue layers were virtually equivalent to ethinyl estradiol, confirming a full estrogen agonist effect [38].

8. What Are the Effects of Ospemifene on Serum Lipids?

Serum lipids, or fats, are principally composed of high-density and low-density lipoproteins (HDL and LDL cholesterol) and triglycerides. Plasma is the complete fluid component of blood, while serum is the remaining fluid portion of the blood after the blood has clotted. Triglycerides are the circulating form of fats consumed in the diet. Levels of serum cholesterol tend to rise following menopause as a result of low levels of circulating estrogen, and high levels of cholesterol, particularly LDL cholesterol, have been associated with the development of cardiovascular disease. The effects of ospemifene on these lipids were evaluated in a pilot study in rhesus macaque monkeys [32].

Over a 15-week period, animals were given ospemifene orally at a high dose weekly for the first three weeks, at a moderate daily dose for the next nine weeks, and then at a low daily dose for the last three weeks. Following weekly dosing for the first three weeks, none of the observed changes in serum lipid concentrations proved to be significant, but the results did show a trend towards increased triglycerides and reduced total and LDL cholesterol, the so-called "bad" cholesterol. After daily dosing for the ensuing nine weeks, the results showed a clear trend towards increasing HDL, the "good" cholesterol, and decreasing triglycerides, total and LDL cholesterol at nine weeks. These trends continued during the final three weeks of dosing, except for triglycerides, which began to rebound after the dose of ospemifene was reduced. Two months after cessation of ospemifene dosing, levels of all serum lipids had returned to near pretreatment levels [32]. In this study, positive downward trends in LDL and total cholesterol were observed, which is in agreement with results seen in clinical trials [50, 51]. An earlier study conducted in rats treated with ospemifene showed a dose-dependent reduction in total serum cholesterol compared to control rats, an effect that was similar to that of raloxifene [31].

Clinical Development

New drugs typically go through three phases of clinical development before an application for approval, called a New Drug Application (NDA), is filed with the FDA. In order to enter human clinical trials, a drug maker must file what is known as an Investigational New Drug (IND) application, which is based on all of the preclinical research performed in animals. Once approved, the IND allows the drug to begin Phase I, which evaluates the safety of a new drug, how it is metabolized by the body, and determines an appropriate dose range for later clinical studies. Phase I studies are typically performed in a small number of volunteers. Phase II studies also involve a relatively small number of subjects and are performed to begin evaluating the efficacy of the selected dose range in the targeted indications. Phase III studies are the largest, longest and most expensive clinical studies to perform. These studies usually involve thousands of patients and are the definitive studies for evaluating the efficacy of a new drug in the treatment of the main targeted indication. If approved drugs of the same type or class are already available for the targeted indication, the new drug must prove to be at least as effective with a favorable side effect profile in order to gain approval. Drug safety continues to be evaluated throughout all phases of clinical development. The odds are very much against a new drug ever getting approved. Out of roughly every 5,000 new compounds that enter development, only one makes it all the way through to FDA approval.

1. Phase I

Two early Phase I studies investigated the safety, tolerability, disposition (pharmacokinetics), and biologic activity (pharmacodynamics) of ospemifene following single and repeated daily oral dosing. The first of these studies involved 28 healthy male volunteers given a single dose of ospemifene at doses ranging from 10 to 800 mg. Results of this initial study showed that ospemifene was well tolerated at doses up to 800 mg and the half-life was approximately 25 hours [52]. A drug's half-life is a measure of how long it takes the body to eliminate half of the drug. The second study involved repeated daily oral dosing of ospemifene for 12 weeks in 40 postmenopausal women at doses ranging from 25 to 200 mg [17, 52]. This was a double-blind, placebo-controlled pilot study, meaning that neither the patients nor their doctors knew whether the study pills contained ospemifene or were a placebo (inactive dummy pill). There were 10 patients at each dose level, two of whom received the placebo and eight of whom received the assigned dose of ospemifene. In addition to side effects and standard laboratory monitoring, the following parameters were evaluated: estrogen-responsive hormonal markers; estrogen-related changes in the endometrium; estrogen-related changes in the vaginal epithelium; and clinical evaluations of vasomotor symptoms (hot flashes). Pharmacokinetic parameters were evaluated after the first dose and after six and 12 weeks of dosing. Pharmacokinetics are measurements of the disposition of a drug within the body, basically how quickly it is absorbed, peak concentrations in the blood, how long it takes to reach the peak concentration, the half-life, and how the drug is ultimately eliminated from the body.

The results of the Phase I pilot study in postmenopausal women showed that ospemifene was well tolerated and did not cause any abnormalities in standard blood, liver, or kidney laboratory tests [17]. At doses above 100 mg/day, significant decreases were seen in follicle-stimulating hormone, indicating that ospemifene was having an estrogenic effect in the pituitary gland, which is located in the brain and releases hormones that regulate the menstrual cycle, but no changes were seen in serum estrogen. Follicle-stimulating hormone stimulates the maturation of ovarian follicles and the production of estrogen in females, and the production of sperm in males. There were no clinically meaningful changes observed with respect to endometrial thickness as assessed by ultrasound at any dose. Only minimal changes in cellular proliferation were seen at doses higher than 100 mg/day, and no endometrial hyperplasia, which is an abnormal, noncancerous increase in cell numbers, was seen at any dose. No significant changes in menopausal symptoms, including hot flashes, sweating, insomnia or headache were observed, but interestingly, there was a tendency for these symptoms to decrease at lower doses and increase at the higher doses. The most notable finding in this study was the consistent and highly significant estrogenic effects on the vaginal epithelium as assessed by the vaginal maturation index (see Chapter 1), which takes into account the percentages of parabasal and superficial cells in the vaginal epithelium [17]. Data from this study showing that the half-life of ospemifene was about 29 hours, coupled with the preclinical data discussed earlier, indicated that the drug could reasonably be given once a day [17, 52], should be given with food [53], and that it is likely to be effective at daily doses of 25-200 mg.

Later Phase I studies were performed to more clearly define ospemifene's metabolism and pharmacokinetics, and how food affects oral bioavailability of the drug [53-57]. Bioavailability is a measure of how much of the dose taken orally actually makes it into the general circulation, making it available to exert the desired effect. While in circulation, ospemifene is highly bound to proteins in the blood plasma (i.e. the fluid component of the blood), and it is extensively metabolized in the liver to form the main metabolite, 4-hydroxyospemifene [54]. Both ospemifene and its metabolite are excreted in the feces, with very small amounts eliminated through the urine. In agreement with the Phase I pilot study in postmenopausal women, the half-life of ospemifene was found to be 29.1 hours [54]. In a study conducted specifically to determine the effect of food on oral bioavailability, giving ospemifene with food caused maximum serum concentrations two to three times that seen when ospemifene was given in the fasted state [53].

2. Phase II

Taken together, data from all of the Phase I studies indicated that the appropriate dose range of ospemifene was between 25 and 100 mg once daily. While higher doses were well tolerated, doses below 100 mg/day avoided some adverse estrogenic side effects while maintaining clear advantageous estrogenic effects, especially in the vaginal epithelium. The ospemifene Phase II development program was designed to assess the efficacy of ospemifene in the selected dose range in as many potential indications as possible, while continuing to evaluate overall safety. Two 12-week Phase II studies were performed in postmenopausal women, the first a double-blind, randomized, placebo-controlled trial, and one in which ospemifene was compared to raloxifene, which as previously mentioned had already been approved for the treatment and prevention of osteoporosis in postmenopausal women.

2.1. Double-Blind, Placebo-Controlled Phase II Study in Postmenopausal Women

The first Phase II study included a total of 160 healthy postmenopausal women who were randomized to receive either a placebo or ospemifene at 30, 60, or 90 mg/day with food [51, 58, 59]. In addition to standard laboratory safety assessments and monitoring of side effects, endometrial safety was carefully monitored by measuring endometrial thickening, microscopic examination of tissue biopsies, and evaluation of cellular proliferation using a special stain [59]. Indicators of potential efficacy included serum triglycerides and cholesterol, vascular (blood vessel) markers for the assessment of cardiovascular treatment potential [51], serum and urinary indicators to assess bone turnover [58], vaginal maturation index to assess vulvar and vaginal atrophy treatment potential, and the Kupperman Index to assess the potential of ospemifene for the treatment of menopausal symptoms [59]. The Kupperman Index is a numerical index that scores 11 different menopausal symptoms, including hot flashes, insomnia, nervousness, vertigo, headache and palpitations. Each symptom is scored on a scale from 0 to 3, with 0 being no symptoms and 3 being the most severe.

2.2. Ospemifene Compared to Raloxifene

The second Phase II study was similar in design to the placebo-controlled study, except that an alternate medication, raloxifene, was used in place of the placebo [50, 60]. As pointed out earlier, when there is an existing medication already approved for the targeted indication, the new drug must prove to be at least equally effective with a favorable side effect profile. Because raloxifene was a SERM already approved for use in treating osteoporosis, ospemifene was compared to raloxifene in this study. At the time this study was conducted, osteoporosis was still one of the targeted indications for ospemifene. This 12-week, double-blind, randomized trial included 118 healthy postmenopausal women treated with either ospemifene (30, 60, or 90 mg/day) or raloxifene (60 mg/day). The goals of this study were to: (1) evaluate the effects of ospemifene compared to raloxifene with respect to hormonal status, serum lipids (cholesterol and triglycerides), genital tract and tolerability in postmenopausal women [50]; and (2) assess the effects of ospemifene on indicators of bone turnover in postmenopausal women compared to raloxifene [60], which was an approved treatment and preventive agent for postmenopausal osteoporosis. Safety and efficacy evaluations in this study were similar to the placebo-controlled Phase II study.

2.3. Phase II Results Summary

In these Phase II studies, ospemifene was again clinically well tolerated, and routine safety assessments indicated no safety issues [50, 59]. Pituitary hormone responses were similar to those seen in the Phase I pilot study, with mild suppression of follicle-stimulating hormone and luteinizing hormone occurring mostly at the 90-mg dose, which is an indicator of estrogenic effects. Luteinizing hormone stimulates ovulation in females and production of testosterone in males. Though the effect was not significant, raloxifene was also found to suppress follicle-stimulating hormone [50, 59]. Assessments of vascular markers and serum cholesterol showed neither clinically beneficial nor adverse effects of ospemifene or raloxifene at any dose level [50, 51]. Both studies revealed that ospemifene had endometrial effects similar to those seen in the Phase I pilot study. Slight thickening and occasional mild proliferative changes in the endometrium were observed, but there was no evidence of hyperplasia or bleeding [50, 59]. Measurements of bone turnover indicators in both Phase II studies showed a clear, dose-dependent reduction in bone turnover. This effect was greatest at the highest dose of ospemifene tested, 90 mg, which was similar to the effect of raloxifene [58, 60]. Because the study population was not restricted to osteoporotic subjects, the magnitude of the changes in bone markers observed in these studies was lower than would have been expected in an osteoporotic population. The impact of ospemifene in the treatment of menopausal symptoms in these studies was mixed. In the placebo-controlled study, no meaningful changes in menopausal symptoms were observed in any group [59], while in the study comparing ospemifene and raloxifene, symptoms decreased in all ospemifene treatment groups. Ospemifene proved better than raloxifene in decreasing menopausal symptoms, particularly at the 60-mg dose [50].

Similar to the Phase I pilot study, the results from these two Phase II studies showed that ospemifene produced significant, beneficial estrogenic effects on the vaginal maturation index. The vaginal maturation index takes into account the percentages of three different cell layers in the vaginal epithelium: parabasal cells (the innermost layer); intermediate cells (the middle layer); and superficial cells (the outermost layer). An effective treatment for vulvar and vaginal atrophy will decrease the number of parabasal cells, which are the most immature, and increase the numbers of intermediate and superficial cells, which are the more mature cell layers. In the placebo-controlled Phase II study, ospemifene had a clear estrogenic effect on the vaginal epithelium at all dose levels as assessed by changes in the percentages of parabasal, intermediate and superficial cells. Parabasal cells decreased significantly, while significant increases in intermediate and superficial cells were observed at all dose levels except for 30 mg, which did not significantly increase superficial cells [59]. In the second Phase II study, ospemifene exerted similar effects on the vaginal epithelium, while no meaningful changes were seen with raloxifene treatment. Significant differences were observed between all doses of ospemifene and raloxifene, except for parabasal cells at the 60-mg dose [50]. Overall results from the Phase I and Phase II studies clearly showed the potential benefits of ospemifene in the treatment of vulvar and vaginal atrophy due to menopause.

3. Phase III

Three potential indications for ospemifene emerged from the Phase I-II studies. The pharmacological similarity of ospemifene to the other approved SERMs and strong animal data made it likely that ospemifene would prove to be effective in the treatment of osteoporosis and breast cancer, but the clinical data generated in the Phase II trials was limited. Because of this and the fact that demonstrating efficacy in breast cancer and osteoporosis is a difficult and time-consuming process, especially since other SERMs for these indications were already approved, the treatment of vulvar and vaginal atrophy was the best indication to target for the Phase III development of ospemifene. The decision to target vulvar and vaginal atrophy was based on the following factors: (1) The clinical data were clear, compelling and consistent with objective clinical indicators such as the vaginal maturation index; (2) There were clear guidelines published by the FDA for the clinical data required to receive approval for the treatment of vulvar and vaginal atrophy. While not all of the clinical parameters needed to obtain FDA approval had been tested in Phase II, the objective parameters that were measured were well correlated with the missing subjective measurements studied with other drugs; (3) The Phase II studies provided evidence that the dose required to treat vulvar and vaginal atrophy would be at the low end of the tested dose range, thus minimizing concerns about side effects; (4) No drug in this class had been approved for the treatment of vulvar and vaginal atrophy, which meant that ospemifene would not have to be compared to any existing medications. All approved treatments for vulvar and vaginal atrophy at the time contained estrogen, which was quickly falling out of favor following publication of the results from the WHI's study of estrogen plus progestin [15]. There was thus an unmet medical need for a non-estrogen alternative; and (5) The number of women suffering from the symptoms of vulvar and vaginal atrophy was very large and underserved by existing products.

The FDA allowed the Phase III development plan for ospemifene to be based on the agency's guidance previously written for estrogen-based products. This guidance specified that a new drug like ospemifene required two 12-week double-blind, placebo-controlled trials in women suffering from moderate to severe vulvar and vaginal atrophy. In addition to routine safety assessments, patients were required to have endometrial biopsies at the beginning and end of the treatment period. Demonstration of efficacy required statistically significant improvement in four different endpoints, including a decrease in parabasal cells, an increase in superficial cells, a decrease in vaginal pH and improvement of the patient's self-identified most bothersome symptom (MBS), which could be vaginal dryness, itching, dysuria, bleeding, or dyspareunia. Each symptom was assessed on a four-point scale specified as none, mild, moderate or severe. In addition to the 12-week efficacy trials, one-year endometrial safety had to be confirmed by an incidence of endometrial hyperplasia of less than 1% after treatment of 100-200 patients for one year at the dose to be marketed.

While the FDA guidance was quite helpful, many questions remained regarding clinical trial design and analysis. Perhaps the most important detail was selection of the dose range. Based on vaginal maturation index data and the safety profile from previous clinical studies, the ospemifene doses selected for the first Phase III study were 30 and 60 mg compared to placebo. The higher 90-mg dose was not studied because it failed to demonstrate any additional efficacy compared to the 60-mg dose in earlier studies. Methods for the analysis of efficacy data were also somewhat unclear. The FDA guidance called for the evaluation of three endpoints, but the vaginal maturation index is actually composed of two components, parabasal and superficial cells of the vaginal epithelium. Although demonstration of statistical significance at four different endpoints posed an unusually difficult obstacle to overcome and is rarely required, the FDA insisted that each of these four endpoints had to be analyzed separately and show statistically significant improvement. Data analysis was further complicated by the various most bothersome symptom categories. Efficacy in alleviating symptoms was by far the most difficult parameter to prove and would dictate the number of subjects needed for each study. The FDA required that the symptomatic data had to be analyzed only for the patients' most bothersome symptom and that each symptom had to be analyzed separately. This necessitated a much larger number of subjects than originally planned because each symptom was essentially a separate efficacy study. Further complicating this situation was the uncertainty about how each most bothersome symptom was distributed within the study population. Another unanticipated study design issue was the FDA requirement that a lubricant be included in all study groups. The final Phase III clinical development plan called for two 12-week efficacy studies and a large one-year endometrial safety study. The two efficacy trials were run sequentially so that design improvements and modifications based on the results of the first study could be incorporated into the second study.

3.1. First Pivotal Phase III Trial

The first Phase III clinical trial of ospemifene included 826 postmenopausal women with symptomatic vulvar and vaginal atrophy [7]. To be included in this study, the subjects must have had less than 5% superficial cells on vaginal smear, a vaginal pH greater than 5 and at least one most bothersome symptom. Patients were randomized to blinded treatment with either placebo or ospemifene (30 or 60 mg/day). After completing 12 weeks of treatment, patients were allowed to enter the long-term safety study (see below). All patients were provided with vaginal lubricant to be used as needed. The four primary endpoints (decrease in parabasal cells, increase in superficial cells, decrease in vaginal pH, and improvement in the patients' most bothersome symptom) were analyzed using methods previously agreed upon with the FDA. Because more than one dose level was employed in the study, efficacy had to be evaluated using a step down approach. Specifically, significance had to be observed at the 60-mg dose before the 30-mg dose could be considered. In the same manner, multiplicity of symptomatic evaluation was addressed with a step down procedure where significance had to be demonstrated in vaginal dryness before dyspareunia could be evaluated. Routine side effect and laboratory assessments were performed as well as endometrial thickness and histology by biopsy. Histology is the evaluation of the microscopic tissue structure.

Ospemifene was well tolerated, and no changes in routine laboratory tests were observed. A high rate of study completion was seen, with 86% of the placebo patients and 80% and 85% of the ospemifene 30-mg and 60-mg patients, respectively, completing the study. Side effects emerging with treatment were similar in all treatment groups. A total of nine patients experienced serious side effects, four in the placebo group, five in the ospemifene 30-mg group, and none at the 60-mg dose. The most common side effect was hot flashes, which were experienced by 3% of the placebo patients, 10% of the patients who received 30 mg ospemifene, and 8% of those who received 60 mg. Very few patients experienced severe hot flashes or discontinued treatment because of hot flashes, but the 30-mg dose did appear to be slightly worse than either the placebo or the 60-mg dose. Urinary tract infections were seen slightly more frequently in the ospemifene-treated women, but this may have been related to a higher frequency of sexual activity. Endometrial thickness differed by less than one millimeter between the three treatment groups at the end of 12 weeks of therapy, and no endometrial hyperplasia was observed in any of the groups. The efficacy of ospemifene was demonstrated unequivocally by all objective measures. Increases in the percentages of superficial cells were significantly greater than placebo at both ospemifene doses (placebo 2%, 30 mg 8%, and 60 mg 11%), and parabasal cells were decreased significantly compared to placebo at both doses (placebo 4%, 30 mg 22%, and 60 mg 30%). Vaginal pH decreased significantly more than placebo in both ospemifene treatment groups (placebo 0.1, 30 mg 0.7, and 60 mg 1.0 pH point) [7].

The two most bothersome symptoms that occurred frequently enough for analysis were dyspareunia (46%) and vaginal dryness (39%). Improvement in these symptoms was positive, particularly at the 60-mg dose. After 12 weeks of treatment, the vaginal dryness symptom score decreased significantly by 1.22 and 1.24 points in the 30-mg and 60-mg groups, respectively, compared to 0.84 points in the placebo group. Ospemifene decreased dyspareunia symptom scores by 1.19 and 1.02 points at the 60-mg and 30-mg doses, respectively. Though the decrease at both doses was more than placebo (0.89), the difference reached significance only at the 60-mg dose. Approximately

30% of the women used lubricant at the beginning of the study. As the study progressed, lubricant use decreased in all groups, with the greatest decrease seen in the active treatment groups [7].

This first pivotal Phase III trial clearly showed that ospemifene was effective in the treatment of symptomatic vulvar and vaginal atrophy even when the use of lubricants was allowed, with a favorable safety profile during the 12 weeks of treatment. Ospemifene 60 mg appeared to be the most effective dose, and it actually had a slightly better clinical profile compared to the 30-mg dose [7].

3.2. Second Pivotal Phase III Trial

Based on the results of the first Phase III study as well as the Phase I-II studies showing inferiority of the 30-mg dose, the second pivotal Phase III study compared 60 mg ospemifene to placebo [9, 10]. As in the first Phase III study, lubricants were issued to all subjects to be used as needed. Since the two vulvar and vaginal atrophy symptoms that occurred frequently enough to be effectively evaluated were vaginal dryness and dyspareunia, these two symptoms were analyzed as two separate studies. The Female Sexual Satisfaction Survey, a standardized scale used to evaluate quality of life improvements, was also included. Other than these differences, the two additional Phase III studies (vaginal dryness [9] and dyspareunia [10]) were identical to the first Phase III study. The two identically designed studies of vaginal dryness and dyspareunia were conducted simultaneously with separate randomization schedules, databases and data analyses. These 12-week studies examined the safety and efficacy of 60 mg ospemifene compared to placebo, with safety and efficacy being evaluated using the same parameters as the first Phase III study.

3.2.1. Dyspareunia Study

In the dyspareunia study, a total of 605 patients were randomized for treatment with either ospemifene 60 mg or placebo given daily for 12 weeks [10]. Ospemifene efficacy was again clearly demonstrated in all four primary endpoints. The decrease in the percentage of parabasal cells, the increase in the percentage of superficial cells, and the decreases in vaginal pH and the severity of dyspareunia symptoms seen with ospemifene treatment were highly significantly different compared to the placebo group, similar to the results from the first Phase III study. As in the first study, the use of a lubricant was similar in the two groups at the beginning of the study and decreased during treatment in both groups, more so in the ospemifene treatment group than the placebo. Ospemifene was again well tolerated, with more ospemifene-treated patients (92%) completing the study than in the placebo group (88%). However, a slightly higher percentage of ospemifene-treated patients (4.6%) discontinued treatment due to side effects compared to the patients receiving the placebo (3.3%). No serious side effects related to treatment were reported in either group. The most frequently encountered side effects in the ospemifene group were hot flashes (6.6% vs. 4.3% for placebo) and urinary tract infections (5.6% vs. 3.6% for placebo). Endometrial thickness increased slightly more in the ospemifene group (0.4 mm) compared to placebo (0.1 mm), but no cases of hyperplasia were observed [10].

3.2.2. Vaginal Dryness Study

In the vaginal dryness study, a total of 314 patients experiencing a most bothersome symptom of moderate to severe vaginal dryness were randomized to treatment with either placebo or 60 mg ospemifene [9]. All three objective measures of efficacy were significantly improved with ospemifene treatment. As in previous studies, the decreases in parabasal cells and vaginal pH and the increase in superficial cells were highly significant compared to the placebo group. For the subjective measure of most bothersome symptom alleviation, the improvement in vaginal dryness was greater in the ospemifene-treated patients (-1.3) than in the placebo group (-1.1), but this difference fell just short of being statistically significant. When the data was analyzed based only on those patients who had completed at least 10 weeks of treatment with a compliance rate of at least 85%, a significantly greater improvement in vaginal dryness symptoms was seen with ospemifene treatment (-1.4) compared to the placebo (-1.1). There were also greater proportions of patients describing either no or mild vaginal dryness (30% vs. 23%) and patients improving by 2-3 levels in their symptom score (50% vs. 34%) in the ospemifene-treated patients compared to those who received placebo. The safety profile in this study was similar to that reported in previous studies. As in the dyspareunia study and the first Phase III study, the most frequently encountered side effects seen with ospemifene treatment were hot flashes and urinary tract infections. Serious side effects were similar in the two groups, but one case of deep vein thrombosis (blood clots) was seen in the ospemifene group that was considered possibly related to treatment. Endometrial thickening was more evident in the ospemifene group compared to placebo, but no cases of endometrial hyperplasia were reported [9].

3.3. Phase III Long-Term Safety Study

As previously discussed, FDA guidance required that 100-200 patients be treated at the intended dose of ospemifene for one year, and endometrial biopsies had to confirm less than a 1% incidence of hyperplasia with a high degree of confidence. Some long-term safety data with endometrial biopsies were obtained from the extension of the first pivotal Phase III study [61, 62], but in order to reach the required one-year exposure, a third Phase III study was initiated looking primarily at long-term safety [8]. This study randomized postmenopausal women with an intact uterus and suffering from vulvar and vaginal atrophy to treatment with either ospemifene 60 mg or placebo daily for 52 weeks using a 6:1 randomization schedule, meaning approximately one-seventh of the patients would receive placebo and six-sevenths would receive ospemifene. Safety assessments included endometrial biopsy, endometrial thickness, and breast and gynecological exams. Efficacy at 12 weeks was also examined with respect to the vaginal maturation index and vaginal pH. Unlike the dyspareunia and vaginal dryness studies, no symptomatic efficacy measures were conducted in this study. A total of 426 patients were randomized to treatment with ospemifene 60 mg (363 patients) or placebo (63 patients). Out of the 349 patients who completed 52 weeks of treatment, there were 294 in the ospemifene group and 55 in the placebo group. Changes in the objective measures of efficacy—decreases in vaginal pH and percentage of parabasal cells, and increase in the percentage of superficial cells in the vaginal epithelium—at 12 weeks of treatment were similar in magnitude to those seen in the previous studies, being highly significant compared to placebo [8]. Safety outcomes are discussed below in the comprehensive safety section (3.5).

3.4. Phase III Efficacy Summary

A summary of ospemifene's efficacy from all of the Phase III clinical trials is presented in Tables 4.2-4.6. In the Tables, the lowercase letter p signifies probability, thus if p<0.05, this means that the probability that the observed result occurred by chance is less than 5%. Normally, for a result to be statistically significant, the p-value must be 0.05 or less. The objective measures were all consistently positive and highly statistically significant in all four Phase III studies. Although changes in these parameters were significant at the 30-mg dose, the magnitude was less than that observed at 60 mg. Parabasal cells decreased 30-40% at the 60-mg dose, with small and inconsistent changes in the placebo group (Table 4.2). Superficial cells increased 5-10% with little if any change in the placebo group (Table 4.3).

Vaginal pH decreased by about one point at the 60-mg dose (Table 4.4). As assessed by these measures, efficacy was maintained through one full year of treatment [8].

Table 4.2. Summary of Ospemifene Efficacy (Phase III): Vaginal Maturation Index (Parabasal Cells of the Vaginal Epithelium)

	Parabasal Cells (%)		
Phase III Trials	Placebo	30 mg	60 mg
First Pivotal			
#Patients	268	280	276
Change[†]	4.0	-21.9*	-30.1*
Second Pivotal (Dyspareunia)			
#Patients	302	—	303
Change[†]	0.0	—	-40.2*
Second Pivotal (Vaginal Dryness)			
#Patients	154	—	160
Change[†]	-3.9	—	-31.7*
Third (Long-Term Safety)			
#Patients	63	—	363
Change[†]	0	—	-40*

*p<0.001 compared to placebo.
[†]Change from baseline to week 12.

Table 4.3. Summary of Ospemifene Efficacy (Phase III): Vaginal Maturation Index (Superficial Cells of the Vaginal Epithelium)

	Superficial Cells (%)		
Phase III Trials	Placebo	30 mg	60 mg
First Pivotal			
#Patients	268	280	276
Change[†]	2.2	7.8*	10.8*
Second Pivotal (Dyspareunia)			
#Patients	302	—	303
Change[†]	1.7	—	12.3*

Phase III Trials	Placebo	30 mg	60 mg
Second Pivotal (Vaginal Dryness)			
#Patients	154	—	160
Change†	0.0	—	7.0*
Third (Long-Term Safety)			
#Patients	63	—	363
Change†	0	—	5*

*p<0.001 compared to placebo.
†Change from baseline to week 12.

Table 4.4. Summary of Ospemifene Efficacy (Phase III): Vaginal pH

	Vaginal pH		
Phase III Trials	Placebo	30 mg	60 mg
First Pivotal			
#Patients	268	280	276
Change†	-0.10	-0.67*	-1.01*
Second Pivotal (Dyspareunia)			
#Patients	302	—	303
Change†	-0.07	—	-0.94*
Second Pivotal (Vaginal Dryness)			
#Patients	154	—	160
Change†	-0.25	—	-0.95*
Third (Long-Term Safety)			
#Patients	63	—	363
Change†	-0.16	—	-1.21*

*p<0.001 compared to placebo.
†Change from baseline to week 12.

With respect to symptomatic relief of the major symptoms of vulvar and vaginal atrophy (i.e. dyspareunia and vaginal dryness) as measured by the four-point scale, ospemifene 60 mg demonstrated superiority compared to placebo and 30 mg ospemifene. For dyspareunia, symptomatic relief was significant at the 60-mg dose in both pivotal Phase III studies (Table 4.5). The 30-mg dose was better than placebo, but the improvement failed to reach statistical significance. The number of patients who experienced an improvement in their symptom score of at least two points was higher with ospemifene 60 mg compared to placebo and ospemifene 30 mg [7].

Table 4.5. Summary of Ospemifene Efficacy (Phase III): Symptoms of VVA (Dyspareunia)

MBS	Treatment Group		
Dyspareunia	Placebo	30 mg	60 mg
First Pivotal			
#Patients	124	136	120
Change from Baseline	-0.89	-1.02	-1.19*
Second Pivotal Dyspareunia			
#Patients	302	—	303
Change from Baseline	-1.2	—	-1.5**

MBS= Most Bothersome Symptom.
*p<0.05 compared to placebo.
**p<0.0001 compared to placebo.

Table 4.6. Summary of Ospemifene Efficacy (Phase III): Symptoms of VVA (Vaginal Dryness)

MBS	Treatment Group		
Vaginal Dryness	Placebo	30 mg	60 mg
First Pivotal			
#Patients	104	102	118
Change from Baseline (ITT)	-0.84	-1.22*	-1.26*
Pivotal Vaginal Dryness			
#Patients	154	—	160
Change from Baseline (ITT)	-1.1	—	-1.3†
Change from Baseline (PP)	-1.1	—	-1.4*
2-3 Level Improvement (ITT)	34.4%	—	46.3%
2-3 Level Improvement (PP)	34.3%	—	50.4%

MBS= Most Bothersome Symptom.
ITT= Intent to Treat.
PP= Per Protocol.
*p<0.05.
†p=0.08.

A recently published review article summarizes all of the available clinical data regarding the efficacy and safety of ospemifene in the treatment of dyspareunia [63].

Symptomatic improvement in patients with vaginal dryness was significantly better at both 30 mg and 60 mg in the first Phase III study [7] (Table 4.6). This was true when measured by either the average on the four-point symptom scale or the number of patients who experienced an improvement of at least two points on the scale. In the second Phase III study, the magnitude of improvement in vaginal dryness was similar, but fell short of being statistically significant when all patients were included (the intent-to-treat population). The difference was significant when the analysis was restricted to those patients that completed at least 10 weeks of treatment (the per protocol population). Other secondary analyses of efficacy in this group such as number of responders, number of patients with two or more levels of improvement and number of patients with complete relief of symptoms all supported the conclusion that vaginal dryness was effectively treated in this study [9].

3.5. Comprehensive Safety Summary

Unlike efficacy, which is best evaluated by considering the results of individual studies that are designed to show clinical effects, safety is better considered as a reflection of total exposures from all studies combined. A total of 1,892 patients were exposed to ospemifene during the Phase II and Phase III studies, with an average duration of exposure of 182 days, the majority of which was at the 60-mg dose. Over 400 patients had in excess of one year of ospemifene treatment. All patients were postmenopausal with an average age of 59 years and 86% were on concomitant medications.

In these studies, no clinically meaningful changes in routine safety assessments, including blood chemistry and urinalysis, were identified. Blood lipid values were favorably impacted with ospemifene treatment. The most common side effects associated with ospemifene 60 mg treatment were hot flashes (7.5% vs. 2.6% placebo), vaginal discharge (3.8% vs. 0.3% placebo), muscle spasms (3.2% vs. 0.9% placebo) and headaches (2.4% vs. 2.4% placebo) [12]. Although vasomotor symptoms were more common in ospemifene-treated patients, these symptoms were well tolerated and rarely led to study discontinuation [8]. Urinary tract infections were also more common in ospemifene-treated patients, especially early in the trials. It has been speculated that this may be related to more frequent sexual activity, meaning that ospemifene was improving symptoms, thus leading to increased sexual activity, but this has not been confirmed [7]. As treatment continued, urinary tract infections seemed to occur at similar rates in both the ospemifene and placebo groups [62]. All serious side effects that emerged during the studies that were not necessarily related to drug treatment were slightly higher in patients treated with 60 mg ospemifene (7.3%) than placebo (5.9%) when evaluated by patient, but lower for ospemifene 60 mg compared to placebo when evaluated by exposure [10]. No deaths occurred during any of the ospemifene trials.

Of particular interest with SERMs is the frequency of cardiovascular events. Six ospemifene-treated patients (0.3%) and one placebo-treated patient (0.1%) discontinued treatment because of a cardiovascular event. These included two cases of deep vein thrombosis (i.e. blood clots), three cerebrovascular accidents (i.e. strokes) and one myocardial infarction (i.e. heart attack) [8, 9, 61]. No cases of thromboembolism (i.e. blood clots clogging blood vessels) were reported. One cardiovascular event occurred in the placebo-treated patients [10]. The incidence of deep vein thrombosis was 0.1%, which is lower than that reported for recently approved SERMs [12]. No electrocardiogram changes were identified in patients taking ospemifene, meaning that ospemifene treatment had no meaningful effects on the heart. A detailed clinical evaluation of the impact of ospemifene required by the FDA was negative.

Endometrial safety was a major point of emphasis during the clinical development of ospemifene. Transvaginal ultrasound before, during and after treatment was used to monitor and detect changes in the endometrium. Compared to placebo, which showed no change, average endometrial thickness increased by less than one millimeter during 52 weeks of treatment with 60 mg ospemifene [8]. The number of patients with endometrial thickening greater than eight millimeters at the end of one year of treatment was higher in ospemifene-treated patients (1%) compared to placebo (0%). No cases of endometrial hyperplasia or endometrial cancer were detected by biopsy at the end of one year of treatment [62]. Although one patient did have a biopsy that showed endometrial hyperplasia three months after the last dose of ospemifene [8], one case in 347 biopsies after one year of treatment is well below the threshold for concern. Five patients treated with 60 mg ospemifene had an endometrial polyp on biopsy (1.4%), only one of which (0.3%) was confirmed to be a true polyp [8]. A polyp is basically a mass of tissue that bulges outward from the normal tissue surface. Bleeding or spotting occurred in 1.4% of patients with an intact uterus treated with ospemifene [62] compared to 0.7% of similar placebo-treated patients [7]. All of the clinical data from the Phase II and Phase III trials regarding the effects of ospemifene on endometrial safety are discussed in an article recently published in the journal *Menopause* [64].

Ospemifene demonstrated a very good breast safety profile. While there were reports of breast tenderness, breast mass and breast pain, the frequency of these events was low and similar to that which occurred in the placebo group [8, 62]. There were two cases of breast cancer reported among the patients treated with placebo, but this is a number to be expected in this population based on the number of patients and the length of treatment. Interestingly, there were no cases of breast cancer observed in the patients treated with ospemifene, which is consistent with all of the preclinical data suggesting that ospemifene is effective in preventing breast cancer [8, 61, 62].

Conclusion

Following completion of the Phase III development program and finalization of the tablet formulation in 2011, a New Drug Application was submitted to the FDA in April of 2012. Ospemifene, which is being sold under the trade name Osphena™ by Shionogi Inc., was approved by the FDA for the treatment of moderate to severe dyspareunia associated with vulvar and vaginal atrophy due to menopause in February of 2013 without the requirement for additional studies, which are typically required for newly approved drugs. Although the FDA did not grant approval for the treatment of vaginal dryness, the close association to vulvar and vaginal atrophy of the symptoms of vaginal dryness and dyspareunia as documented by objective criteria and multiple parameter analyses that support efficacy in the treatment of vaginal dryness, there is little doubt that ospemifene is an effective treatment for vaginal dryness associated with vulvar and vaginal atrophy due to menopause.

The FDA required that the ospemifene label contain a boxed warning similar to estrogen products [12], a warning considered unwarranted by some [65]. It is our opinion that the FDA decided on this labeling out of an abundance of caution rather than sound scientific evidence. While ospemifene does have a very slight estrogenic effect on the endometrium, both preclinical and clinical data clearly show that this effect is not anywhere near the magnitude of that of estrogen. In fact, ospemifene's effects are much more similar to those of the SERM raloxifene, which does not have the same boxed warning on its labeling. More pointedly, as discussed earlier in this Chapter, ospemifene is actually one of the metabolites of toremifene, a SERM approved for the treatment of breast cancer. The labeling for toremifene does not include a boxed warning for estrogenic effects on the endometrium. Ospemifene is a synthetic, non-steroidal, non-estrogen SERM and should be labeled in a manner consistent with other SERMs and with the available clinical data. To compare ospemifene to Premarin®, which is a product containing many different estrogens as well as numerous unknown steroids is illogical and akin to comparing apples and oranges. This labeling controversy is discussed in greater detail in Chapters 2 and 5.

The current ospemifene label also suggests that ospemifene should not be used in women who have or may develop breast cancer. While it is true that the currently available clinical data are inadequate to make any claim that ospemifene has beneficial effects in the treatment or prevention of breast cancer, there are no clinical data showing that ospemifene would increase risk in these patients either. In fact, virtually all data generated to date suggest that ospemifene, similar to other FDA-approved SERMs, acts as an antiestrogen in the breast and is more likely to have beneficial than detrimental effects [42]. Phase IV clinical trials, which are conducted after a drug has already been approved to demonstrate efficacy in additional indications, of ospemifene in postmenopausal women at high risk for the development of breast cancer are being considered. This is discussed in greater detail in Chapter 7.

References

[1]   Bernstein, L., Deapen, D., Cerhan, J. R., Schwartz, S. M., Liff, J., McGann-Maloney, E., et al. (1999). Tamoxifen therapy for breast cancer and endometrial cancer risk. *J Natl Cancer Inst, 91(19)*, 1654-1662.

[2]   Delmas, P. D., Bjarnason, N. H., Mitlak, B. H., Ravoux, A. C., Shah, A. S., Huster, W. J., et al. (1997). Effects of raloxifene on bone mineral density, serum cholesterol concentrations, and uterine endometrium in postmenopausal women. *N Engl J Med, 337(23)*, 1641-1647.

[3]   Jordan, V. C. (2003). Antiestrogens and selective estrogen receptor modulators as multifunctional medicines. 2. Clinical considerations and new agents. *J Med Chem, 46(7)*, 1081-1111.

[4]   Albertazzi, P., Sharma, S. (2005). Urogenital effects of selective estrogen receptor modulators: a systematic review. *Climacteric, 8(3)*, 214-220.

[5]   Jordan, V. C. (2003). Antiestrogens and selective estrogen receptor modulators as multifunctional medicines. 1. Receptor interactions. *J Med Chem, 46(6)*, 883-908.

[6]   Vogel, V. G., Costantino, J. P., Wickerham, D. L., Cronin, W. M., Cecchini, R. S., Atkins, J. N., et al. (2006). Effects of tamoxifen vs raloxifene on the risk of developing invasive breast cancer and other disease outcomes: the NSABP Study of Tamoxifen and Raloxifene (STAR) P-2 trial. *JAMA, 295(23)*, 2727-2741.

[7]   Bachmann, G. A., Komi, J. O. (2010). Ospemifene effectively treats vulvovaginal atrophy in postmenopausal women: results from a pivotal phase 3 study. *Menopause, 17(3)*, 480-486.

[8]   Goldstein, S. R., Bachmann, G. A., Koninckx, P. R., Lin, V. H., Portman, D. J., Ylikorkala, O. (2014). Ospemifene 12-month safety and efficacy in postmenopausal women with vulvar and vaginal atrophy. *Climacteric, 17(2)*, 173-182.

[9]   Portman, D., Palacios, S., Nappi, R. E., Mueck, A. O. (2014). Ospemifene, a non-oestrogen selective oestrogen receptor modulator for the treatment of vaginal dryness associated with postmenopausal vulvar and vaginal atrophy: A randomised, placebo-controlled, phase III trial. *Maturitas, 78(2)*, 91-98.

[10]   Portman, D. J., Bachmann, G. A., Simon, J. A. (2013). Ospemifene, a novel selective estrogen receptor modulator for treating dyspareunia associated with postmenopausal vulvar and vaginal atrophy. *Menopause, 20(6)*, 623-630.

[11]   Lorizio, W., Wu, A. H., Beattie, M. S., Rugo, H., Tchu, S., Kerlikowske, K., et al. (2012). Clinical and biomarker predictors of side effects from tamoxifen. *Breast Cancer Res Treat, 132(3)*, 1107-1118.

[12]   Osphena™ (ospemifene) Prescribing Information. Florham Park, New Jersey: Shionogi Inc.; 2013.

[13]   Chlebowski, R. T., Anderson, G. L., Gass, M., Lane, D. S., Aragaki, A. K., Kuller, L. H., et al. (2010). Estrogen plus progestin and breast cancer incidence and mortality in postmenopausal women. *JAMA, 304(15)*, 1684-1692.

[14]   Nelson, H. D., Walker, M., Zakher, B., Mitchell, J. (2012). Menopausal hormone therapy for the primary prevention of chronic conditions: a

systematic review to update the U.S. Preventive Services Task Force recommendations. *Ann Intern Med, 157(2)*, 104-113.

[15] Rossouw, J. E., Anderson, G. L., Prentice, R. L., LaCroix, A. Z., Kooperberg, C., Stefanick, M. L., et al. (2002). Risks and benefits of estrogen plus progestin in healthy postmenopausal women: principal results From the Women's Health Initiative randomized controlled trial. *JAMA, 288(3)*, 321-333.

[16] Rozenberg, S., Vandromme, J., Antoine, C. (2013). Postmenopausal hormone therapy: risks and benefits. *Nat Rev Endocrinol, 9(4)*, 216-227.

[17] Voipio, S. K., Komi, J., Kangas, L., Halonen, K., DeGregorio, M. W., Erkkola, R. U. (2002). Effects of ospemifene (FC-1271a) on uterine endometrium, vaginal maturation index, and hormonal status in healthy postmenopausal women. *Maturitas, 43(3)*, 207-214.

[18] Osborne, C. K., Wiebe, V. J., McGuire, W. L., Ciocca, D. R., DeGregorio, M. W. (1992). Tamoxifen and the isomers of 4-hydroxytamoxifen in tamoxifen-resistant tumors from breast cancer patients. *J Clin Oncol, 10(2)*, 304-310.

[19] Wiebe, V. J., Osborne, C. K., McGuire, W. L., DeGregorio, M. W. (1992). Identification of estrogenic tamoxifen metabolite(s) in tamoxifen-resistant human breast tumors. *J Clin Oncol, 10(6)*, 990-994.

[20] Bonewald, L. F. (1994). Effects of Estrogen on Growth Factors in Bone. In: R. Ziegler, J. Pfeilschifter, M. Bräutigam, (Eds.), *Sex Steroids and Bone*, pp. 71-94. New York: Springer-Verlag.

[21] DeGregorio, M., Wiebe, V., Kangas, L., Härkönen, P., Väänänen, K., Laine, A., inventors; Orion-Yhtymä Oy, assignee. Triphenylethylenes Compositions (United States Patent). United States of America patent Patent number 5,912,273. 1999.

[22] Shibutani, S., Ravindernath, A., Terashima, I., Suzuki, N., Laxmi, Y. R. Kanno, Y., et al. (2001). Mechanism of lower genotoxicity of toremifene compared with tamoxifen. *Cancer Res, 61(10)*, 3925-3931.

[23] Dahlman-Wright, K., Cavailles, V., Fuqua, S. A., Jordan, V. C. Katzenellenbogen, J. A., Korach, K. S., et al. (2006). International Union of Pharmacology. LXIV. Estrogen receptors. *Pharmacol Rev, 58(4)* 773-781.

[24] Heldring, N., Pike, A., Andersson, S., Matthews, J., Cheng, G., Hartman J., et al. (2007). Estrogen receptors: how do they signal and what are their targets. *Physiol Rev, 87(3)*, 905-931.

[25] Musa, M. A., Khan, M. O., Cooperwood, J. S. (2007). Medicinal chemistry and emerging strategies applied to the development of

selective estrogen receptor modulators (SERMs). *Curr Med Chem*, *14(11)*, 1249-1261.

[26] Brzozowski, A. M., Pike, A. C., Dauter, Z., Hubbard, R. E., Bonn, T., Engstrom, O., et al. (1997). Molecular basis of agonism and antagonism in the oestrogen receptor. *Nature*, *389(6652)*, 753-758.

[27] Feng, W., Ribeiro, R. C., Wagner, R. L., Nguyen, H., Apriletti, J. W., Fletterick, R. J., et al. (1998). Hormone-dependent coactivator binding to a hydrophobic cleft on nuclear receptors. *Science*, *280(5370)*, 1747-1749.

[28] Shang, Y., Brown, M. (2002). Molecular determinants for the tissue specificity of SERMs. *Science*, *295(5564)*, 2465-2468.

[29] Hellmann-Blumberg, U., Taras, T. L., Wurz, G. T., DeGregorio, M. W. (2000). Genotoxic effects of the novel mixed antiestrogen FC-1271a in comparison to tamoxifen and toremifene. *Breast Cancer Res Treat*, *60(1)*, 63-70.

[30] Hellmann-Blumberg, U., Cartner, M. G., Wurz, G. T., DeGregorio, M. W. (1998). Intrinsic reactivity of tamoxifen and toremifene metabolites with DNA. *Breast Cancer Res Treat*, *50(2)*, 135-141.

[31] Qu, Q., Zheng, H., Dahllund, J., Laine, A., Cockcroft, N., Peng, Z., et al. (2000). Selective estrogenic effects of a novel triphenylethylene compound, FC1271a, on bone, cholesterol level, and reproductive tissues in intact and ovariectomized rats. *Endocrinology*, *141(2)*, 809-820.

[32] Wurz, G. T., Hellmann-Blumberg, U., DeGregorio, M. W. (2008). Pharmacologic effects of ospemifene in rhesus macaques: a pilot study. *Basic Clin Pharmacol Toxicol*, *102(6)*, 552-558.

[33] Qu, Q., Harkonen, P. L., Vaananen, H. K. (1999). Comparative effects of estrogen and antiestrogens on differentiation of osteoblasts in mouse bone marrow culture. *J Cell Biochem*, *73(4)*, 500-507.

[34] Michael, H., Harkonen, P. L., Kangas, L., Vaananen, H. K., Hentunen, T. A. (2007). Differential effects of selective oestrogen receptor modulators (SERMs) tamoxifen, ospemifene and raloxifene on human osteoclasts in vitro. *Br J Pharmacol*, *151(3)*, 384-395.

[35] Kallio, A., Guo, T., Lamminen, E., Seppanen, J., Kangas, L., Vaananen, H. K., et al. (2008). Estrogen and the selective estrogen receptor modulator (SERM) protection against cell death in estrogen receptor alpha and beta expressing U2OS cells. *Mol Cell Endocrinol*, *289(1-2)*, 38-48.

[36]   Kangas, L., Harkonen, P., Vaananen, K., Peng, Z. (2014). Effects of the selective estrogen receptor modulator ospemifene on bone in rats. *Horm Metab Res*, *46(1)*, 27-35.

[37]   Taras, T. L., Wurz, G. T., DeGregorio, M. W. (2001). In vitro and in vivo biologic effects of Ospemifene (FC-1271a) in breast cancer. *J Steroid Biochem Mol Biol*, *77(4-5)*, 271-279.

[38]   Unkila, M., Kari, S., Yatkin, E., Lammintausta, R. (2013). Vaginal effects of ospemifene in the ovariectomized rat preclinical model of menopause. *J Steroid Biochem Mol Biol*, *138*, 107-115.

[39]   Kangas, L., Unkila, M. (2013). Tissue selectivity of ospemifene: Pharmacologic profile and clinical implications. *Steroids*, *78(12-13)*, 1273-1280.

[40]   Kangas, L., Harkonen, P., Vaananen, K., Keskitalo, J., Eigeliene, N. (2014). Effects of ospemifene on breast tissue morphology and proliferation: a comparative study versus other selective estrogen receptor modulators in ovariectomized rats. *Horm Metab Res*, *46(5)*, 328-332.

[41]   Soe, L. H., Wurz, G. T., Kao, C. J., Degregorio, M. W. (2013). Ospemifene for the treatment of dyspareunia associated with vulvar and vaginal atrophy: potential benefits in bone and breast. *Int J Womens Health*, *5*, 605-611.

[42]   Wurz, G. T., Soe, L. H., Degregorio, M. W. (2013). Ospemifene, vulvovaginal atrophy, and breast cancer. *Maturitas*, *74(3)*, 220-225.

[43]   Wurz, G. T., Read, K. C., Marchisano-Karpman, C., Gregg, J. P., Beckett, L. A., Yu, Q., et al. (2005). Ospemifene inhibits the growth of dimethylbenzanthracene-induced mammary tumors in Sencar mice. *J Steroid Biochem Mol Biol*, *97(3)*, 230-240.

[44]   Lin, E. Y., Jones, J. G., Li, P., Zhu, L., Whitney, K. D., Muller, W. J., et al. (2003). Progression to malignancy in the polyoma middle T oncoprotein mouse breast cancer model provides a reliable model for human diseases. *Am J Pathol*, *163(5)*, 2113-2126.

[45]   Namba, R., Young, L. J., Maglione, J. E., McGoldrick, E. T., Liu, S., Wurz, G. T., et al. (2005). Selective estrogen receptor modulators inhibit growth and progression of premalignant lesions in a mouse model of ductal carcinoma in situ. *Breast Cancer Res*, *7(6)*, R881-889.

[46]   Burich, R. A., Mehta, N. R., Wurz, G. T., McCall, J. L., Greenberg, B. E., Bell, K. E., et al. (2012). Ospemifene and 4-hydroxyospemifene effectively prevent and treat breast cancer in the MTag.Tg transgenic mouse model. *Menopause*, *19(1)*, 96-103.

[47] Guy, C. T., Cardiff, R. D., Muller, W. J. (1992). Induction of mammary tumors by expression of polyomavirus middle T oncogene: a transgenic mouse model for metastatic disease. *Mol Cell Biol, 12(3)*, 954-961.

[48] Pinkerton, J. V., Goldstein, S. R. (2010). Endometrial safety: a key hurdle for selective estrogen receptor modulators in development. *Menopause, 17(3)*, 642-653.

[49] Zheng, H., Kangas, L., Harkonen, P. L. (2004). Comparative study of the short-term effects of a novel selective estrogen receptor modulator, ospemifene, and raloxifene and tamoxifen on rat uterus. *J Steroid Biochem Mol Biol, 88(2)*, 143-156.

[50] Komi, J., Lankinen, K. S., Harkonen, P., DeGregorio, M. W., Voipio, S., Kivinen, S., et al. (2005). Effects of ospemifene and raloxifene on hormonal status, lipids, genital tract, and tolerability in postmenopausal women. *Menopause, 12(2)*, 202-209.

[51] Ylikorkala, O., Cacciatore, B., Halonen, K., Lassila, R., Lammintausta, R., Rutanen, E. M., et al. (2003). Effects of ospemifene, a novel SERM, on vascular markers and function in healthy, postmenopausal women. *Menopause, 10(5)*, 440-447.

[52] DeGregorio, M. W., Wurz, G. T., Taras, T. L., Erkkola, R. U., Halonen, K. H., Huupponen, R. K. (2000). Pharmacokinetics of (deaminohydroxy)toremifene in humans: a new, selective estrogen-receptor modulator. *Eur J Clin Pharmacol, 56(6-7)*, 469-475.

[53] Koskimies, P., Katila, K., Lammintausta, R., Aaltonen, A. M., Vuorinen, J., Saarni, O., et al. (2013). Oral bioavailability of ospemifene improves with food intake. *Int J Clin Pharmacol Ther, 51(10)*, 787-794.

[54] Koskimies, P., Turunen, J., Lammintausta, R., Scheinin, M. (2013). Single-dose and steady-state pharmacokinetics of ospemifene, a selective estrogen receptor modulator, in postmenopausal women. *Int J Clin Pharmacol Ther, 51(11)*, 861-867.

[55] Lehtinen, T., Tolonen, A., Turpeinen, M., Uusitalo, J., Vuorinen, J., Lammintausta, R., et al. (2013). Effects of cytochrome P450 inhibitors and inducers on the metabolism and pharmacokinetics of ospemifene. *Biopharm Drug Dispos, 34(7)*, 387-395.

[56] Tolonen, A., Koskimies, P., Turpeinen, M., Uusitalo, J., Lammintausta, R., Pelkonen, O. (2013). Ospemifene metabolism in humans in vitro and in vivo: metabolite identification, quantitation, and CYP assignment of major hydroxylations. *Drug Metabol Drug Interact, 28(3)*, 153-161.

[57] Turpeinen, M., Uusitalo, J., Lehtinen, T., Kailajarvi, M., Pelkonen, O., Vuorinen, J., et al. (2013). Effects of ospemifene on drug metabolism

mediated by cytochrome P450 enzymes in humans in vitro and in vivo. *Int J Mol Sci, 14(7)*, 14064-14075.

[58] Komi, J., Heikkinen, J., Rutanen, E. M., Halonen, K., Lammintausta, R., Ylikorkala, O. (2004). Effects of ospemifene, a novel SERM, on biochemical markers of bone turnover in healthy postmenopausal women. *Gynecol Endocrinol, 18(3)*, 152-158.

[59] Rutanen, E. M., Heikkinen, J., Halonen, K., Komi, J., Lammintausta, R., Ylikorkala, O. (2003). Effects of ospemifene, a novel SERM, on hormones, genital tract, climacteric symptoms, and quality of life in postmenopausal women: a double-blind, randomized trial. *Menopause, 10(5)*, 433-439.

[60] Komi, J., Lankinen, K. S., DeGregorio, M., Heikkinen, J., Saarikoski, S., Tuppurainen, M., et al. (2006). Effects of ospemifene and raloxifene on biochemical markers of bone turnover in postmenopausal women. *J Bone Miner Metab, 24(4)*, 314-318.

[61] Simon, J., Portman, D., Mabey, R. G., Jr. (2014). Long-term safety of ospemifene (52-week extension) in the treatment of vulvar and vaginal atrophy in hysterectomized postmenopausal women. *Maturitas, 77(3)*, 274-281.

[62] Simon, J. A., Lin, V. H., Radovich, C., Bachmann, G. A. (2013). One-year long-term safety extension study of ospemifene for the treatment of vulvar and vaginal atrophy in postmenopausal women with a uterus. *Menopause, 20(4)*, 418-427.

[63] Cui, Y., Zong, H., Yan, H., Li, N., Zhang, Y. (2014). The efficacy and safety of ospemifene in treating dyspareunia associated with postmenopausal vulvar and vaginal atrophy: a systematic review and meta-analysis. *J Sex Med, 11(2)*, 487-497.

[64] Constantine, G. D., Goldstein, S. R., Archer, D. F. (2014). Endometrial safety of ospemifene: results of the phase 2/3 clinical development program. *Menopause*;DOI: 10.1097/GME.0000000000000275.

[65] Goldstein, S. R. (2013). Postmenopausal dyspareunia: has the Food and Drug Administration really helped? *Menopause, 20(6)*, 596-597.

Chapter 5

Understanding Side Effects: Boxed Warnings and Package Inserts

Abstract

The U.S. Food and Drug Administration (FDA) enforces strict rules regarding the testing of all prescription therapies prior to their approval for sale to the public. Once the risks and side effects of a therapy have been determined and the FDA has approved it for sale, each prescription is required to be accompanied by a "package insert" which details all of the relevant study results regarding the effectiveness of the product in treating the targeted indication as well as known risks and side effects. In addition, the FDA will require a "boxed warning" on the packaging label when there are risks of serious side effects. In the case of Osphena™ (ospemifene), the FDA has also required that its boxed warning and package insert contain information about potential risks that have not been proven but that might be possible. Because the FDA has chosen to assume that this newer therapy could behave similarly to Premarin® (conjugated equine estrogens), an older therapy with known long-term risks, Osphena™ will be labeled with the same risk profile as the older therapy until long-term studies prove otherwise. While this "guilty until proven innocent" form of conservative labeling is intended to protect the public, we believe that the result is the creation of unnecessary fears of risks and side effects that might likely never occur.

Introduction

Just about every medication that you consume during your lifetime will carry with it both intended and unintended effects on your body. Whether taken as a tablet, capsule, liquid or cream, chemical compounds enter your bloodstream, which sends the medication throughout your body where many different interactions can occur. Some of these interactions have positive effects on the body, and some of them have negative effects. In addition, each individual will react to a given medication slightly differently; on occasion some individuals might react significantly differently. This is precisely why the U.S. Food and Drug Administration (FDA) enforces strict rules regarding the testing of all prescription therapies prior to their approval for sale to the public.

Even compounds as common as aspirin have known side effects that can cause significant health problems. Aside from its intended effects of temporarily reducing pain, inflammation and fever, aspirin has been known to cause stomach bleeding in some individuals, with a higher incidence occurring in people who are age 60 or older. Okay, so should you avoid aspirin in favor of acetaminophen (also known as Tylenol), which is another commonly used pain reducer? Well, acetaminophen has been known to cause severe liver damage, particularly if more than three doses are consumed within a 24-hour period. Does this mean that you should avoid pain killers altogether? Absolutely not. What this means is that it is in your best interest to understand the risks of a medication and consider its alternatives, so that you can choose the one that is best suited for your individual needs.

To help you understand the potential unintended effects of a medication, the FDA requires each prescription to be accompanied by a "package insert" which details all of the relevant study results regarding the effectiveness of the medication in treating the targeted indication as well as the known risks and side effects. The FDA will also require a "boxed warning" on the packaging label when there are risks of serious side effects. Boxed warnings and package inserts, while intended to be helpful, can unfortunately be quite daunting as they typically highlight remote chances of severe side effects, and they commonly contain thousands of words, mainly in technical medical jargon. Let's take time now to review the warnings for Premarin® Vaginal Cream and Osphena™ oral tablets.

Boxed Warnings

A boxed warning specifically highlights any severe health risks that should be understood and accepted prior to administering a medication. It is the strongest warning that you will find on a prescription, which the FDA requires for any medication that has the potential to induce severe adverse effects. Below is the complete boxed warning for Premarin® Vaginal Cream [1].

Premarin® (conjugated estrogens) Vaginal Cream – boxed warning

---

WARNING: ENDOMETRIAL CANCER, CARDIOVASCULAR DISORDERS, BREAST CANCER and PROBABLE DEMENTIA

<u>Estrogen-Alone Therapy</u>

Endometrial Cancer

There is an increased risk of endometrial cancer in a woman with a uterus who uses unopposed estrogens. Adding a progestin to estrogen therapy has been shown to reduce the risk of endometrial hyperplasia, which may be a precursor to endometrial cancer. Adequate diagnostic measures, including directed or random endometrial sampling when indicated, should be undertaken to rule out malignancy in postmenopausal women with undiagnosed persistent or recurring abnormal genital bleeding *[see Warnings and Precautions (5.3)]*.

Cardiovascular Disorders and Probable Dementia

Estrogen-alone therapy should not be used for the prevention of cardiovascular disease or dementia *[see Warnings and Precautions (5.2, 5.4), and Clinical Studies (14.2, 14.3)]*

The Women's Health Initiative (WHI) estrogen-alone substudy reported increased risks of stroke and deep vein thrombosis (DVT) in postmenopausal women (50 to 79 years of age) during 7.1 years of treatment with daily oral conjugated estrogens (CE) [0.625 mg]-alone, relative to placebo *[see Warnings and Precautions (5.2), and Clinical Studies (14.2)]*.

The WHI Memory Study (WHIMS) estrogen-alone ancillary study of the WHI reported an increased risk of developing probable dementia in postmenopausal women 65 years of age or older during 5.2 years of treatment with daily CE (0.625 mg)-alone, relative to placebo. It is unknown whether this finding applies to younger postmenopausal women *[see Warnings and Precautions (5.4), Use in Specific Populations (8.5), and Clinical Studies (14.3)]*.

In the absence of comparable data, these risks should be assumed to be similar for other doses of CE and other dosage forms of estrogens.

Estrogens with or without progestins should be prescribed at the lowest effective doses and for the shortest duration consistent with treatment goals and risks for the individual woman.

Estrogen Plus Progestin Therapy

Cardiovascular Disorders and Probable Dementia

Estrogen plus progestin therapy should not be used for the prevention of cardiovascular disease or dementia *[see Warnings and Precautions (5.2, 5.4), and Clinical Studies (14.2, 14.3)]*.

The WHI estrogen plus progestin substudy reported increased risks of DVT, pulmonary embolism (PE), stroke and myocardial infarction (MI) in postmenopausal women (50 to 79 years of age) during 5.6 years of treatment with daily oral CE (0.625 mg) combined with medroxyprogesterone acetate (MPA) [2.5 mg], relative to placebo *[see Warnings and Precautions (5.2), and Clinical Studies (14.2)]*.

The WHIMS estrogen plus progestin ancillary study of the WHI reported an increased risk of developing probable dementia in postmenopausal women 65 years of age or older during 4 years of treatment with daily CE (0.625 mg) combined with MPA (2.5 mg), relative to placebo. It is unknown whether this finding applies to younger postmenopausal women *[see Warnings and Precautions (5.4), Use in Specific Populations (8.5), and Clinical Studies (14.3)]*.

Breast Cancer

The WHI estrogen plus progestin substudy also demonstrated an increased risk of invasive breast cancer *[see Warnings and Precautions (5.3), and Clinical Studies (14.3)]*.

In the absence of comparable data, these risks should be assumed to be similar for other doses of CE and MPA, and other combinations and dosage forms of estrogens and progestins.

Estrogens with or without progestins should be prescribed at the lowest effective doses and for the shortest duration consistent with treatment goals and risks for the individual woman.

The first thing that you should notice in bold, capitalized type is the warning for endometrial cancer, cardiovascular disorders, breast cancer, and probable dementia. The FDA is highlighting that the use of Premarin® Vaginal Cream could cause any of these severe health problems. Interestingly, below the initial warning, the rest of the box is split into two sections: "Estrogen-Alone Therapy" and "Estrogen Plus Progestin Therapy". The reason for this is that studies have revealed different health issues depending on whether Premarin® is taken alone or in combination with a progestin (a steroid hormone used to protect the uterus) [2-5]. When taken alone, the FDA warns that Premarin® Vaginal Cream increases the risk of developing endometrial cancer if you have a uterus. It also warns of an increased risk of stroke and deep vein thrombosis (i.e. blood clots) in postmenopausal women ages 50-79, as well as an increased risk of probable dementia in postmenopausal women 65 years or older [1].

To reduce the risk of developing endometrial cancer in postmenopausal women with a uterus, Premarin® is frequently prescribed in combination with a progestin [6]. Unfortunately, while reducing the incidence of endometrial cancer, this combination therapy actually increases the risk of developing breast cancer [3]. In addition, studies have revealed that it also increases the risk of deep vein thrombosis, pulmonary embolism (i.e. blockage of a main artery in the lungs), stroke and myocardial infarction (i.e. heart attack) in postmenopausal women aged 50-79 [3]. Furthermore, the risk of developing dementia (e.g. Alzheimer's disease) is not reduced by adding a progestin to the therapy [5].

How can the FDA confidently make these claims of increased health risks, either from Premarin® alone or in combination with a progestin? Well, you might have noticed throughout the boxed warning that the FDA cites several sections of the package insert. This is where we can learn about the substantive information that backs up the warnings. We will review the package insert later, but first let's take a look at the Osphena™ boxed warning [7].

Osphena™ (ospemifene) tablets, for oral use – boxed warning

WARNING: ENDOMETRIAL CANCER AND CARDIOVASCULAR DISORDERS

Endometrial Cancer

OSPHENA is an estrogen agonist/antagonist with tissue selective effects. In the endometrium, OSPHENA has estrogen agonistic effects. There is an increased risk of endometrial cancer in a woman with a uterus who uses unopposed estrogens. Adding a progestin to estrogen therapy reduces the risk of endometrial hyperplasia, which may be a precursor to endometrial cancer. Adequate diagnostic measures, including directed and random endometrial sampling when indicated, should be undertaken to rule out malignancy in postmenopausal women with undiagnosed persistent or recurring abnormal genital bleeding *[see warnings and Precautions (5.2)]*.

Cardiovascular Disorders
There is a reported increased risk of stroke and deep vein thrombosis (DVT) in postmenopausal women (50-79 years of age) who received daily oral conjugated estrogens (CE) [0.625 mg]-alone therapy over 7.1 years as part of the Women's Health Initiative (WHI) *[see Warnings and Precautions (5.1)]*.

In the clinical trials for OSPHENA (duration of treatment up to 15 months), the incidence rates of thromboembolic and hemorrhagic stroke were 0.72 and 1.45 per thousand women, respectively in OSPHENA 60 mg treatment group and 1.04 and 0 in placebo *[see Warnings and Precautions (5.1)]*. The incidence of DVT was 1.45 per thousand women in OSPHENA 60 mg treatment group and 1.04 per thousand women in placebo [see Warnings and Precautions (5.1)]. OSPHENA should be prescribed for the shortest duration consistent with treatment goals and risks for the individual woman.

The Osphena™ boxed warning also begins with bold, capitalized type but it highlights only endometrial cancer and cardiovascular disorders. Then, as you read through the details of the endometrial cancer warning, the FDA cites an increased risk of developing endometrial cancer when using *estrogens*. But wait... Osphena™ is not an estrogen. It is a selective estrogen receptor modulator (SERM), which means that it acts like estrogen in some tissues and is neutral or opposes the action of estrogen in other tissues. No clinical studies have shown that Osphena™ increases the risk of developing endometrial cancer [8-13]. This is a very important point, because we believe that the FDA is mistakenly acting with an overabundance of caution when applying an estrogen-specific warning to a non-estrogen therapy [14]. Why is this a mistake? Because when one therapy is known to increase the risk of developing endometrial cancer, and a different therapy is merely assumed to have the same risk, a woman is left to believe that both therapies carry the same risk. Though the intention might be extra safety, the result could be a therapy choice that actually poses a greater risk.

As you read through the cardiovascular disorder warnings for Osphena™, you will notice yet another warning for women who receive estrogens. There is a reported increased risk of blood clots from a study in postmenopausal women who received daily oral *conjugated estrogens* [2]. These women did not receive a SERM, and they did not receive Osphena™. Again, we believe that this warning is misleading.

Osphena™ is a metabolite (i.e. a by-product of another compound that appears in the body when it is processed by the liver) of another FDA-approved SERM called toremifene, which is sold under the trade name Fareston®. Toremifene is a non-estrogen that is used for the treatment of certain breast cancers in postmenopausal women. Toremifene has been available to the public since 1997 and it carries no warnings for endometrial cancer, stroke, or deep vein thrombosis [15]. To reiterate, Osphena™ is a non-estrogen and it is a major metabolite of toremifene. If the FDA has concerns about potential long-term risks of Osphena™ and it believes that these risks may not surface for years to come, why is the FDA labeling Osphena™ with estrogen-specific warnings instead of toremifene-specific warnings? The logic is elusive.

We are not trying to say that Osphena™ is a miracle drug. Every medication has side effects, and Osphena™ is not unique in that regard. An increased risk of some cardiovascular disorders was, in fact, identified during Phase III clinical trials of Osphena™ [9, 10, 12]. These risks include stroke and blood clots. Similar to the Premarin® Vaginal Cream boxed warning, sections of the package insert are referenced for more information. To understand the magnitude of these Osphena™ risks, as well as those of Premarin® Vaginal Cream, let us now review their respective package inserts.

Package Inserts

Also known as "prescribing information" or "physician labeling", a package insert is commonly found as a multipage pamphlet that accompanies a prescription. In 2006, The FDA issued strict regulations regarding the content and format of prescribing information for medications. Known more formally as the Physician Labeling Rule (PLR) [16], the FDA's intent is to *"enhance the safe and effective use of prescription drug products by providing health care providers with clear and concise prescribing information that is easier to access, read, and use."* As a result, today's package inserts include all of the comprehensive and critical information required for prescribing a medication. The format of all package inserts is consistent, regardless of the medication. Below is a list and description of each section of the full prescribing information found in a package insert. An index of the contents of the package inserts for Premarin® Vaginal Cream and Osphena™ can be found at the end of this Chapter in Tables 5.7 and 5.8.

Standard Package Insert Contents

1. *Indications and usage.* A list of the conditions that the medication is intended to treat.
2. *Dosage and administration.* An explanation of the appropriate dosing ranges and administration methods.
3. *Dosage forms and strengths.* A summary of all available dosage forms and strengths.
4. *Contraindications.* A list of the pre-conditions that should preclude a patient from using the medication.
5. *Warnings and precautions.* A discussion of the risks of developing new health problems from taking the medication.
6. *Adverse reactions.* A list of common side effects that can be experienced while taking the medication.

7. *Drug interactions*. A summary of drugs or foods that may adversely interact with the medication.

8. *Use in specific populations*. A discussion of important differences in response, or recommendations for use, in different types of individuals.

9. *Drug abuse and dependence*. A discussion of the impact that prolonged use can have regarding dependence (omitted if inapplicable).

10. *Overdosage*. A description of the impacts from overdosage, along with a recommendation for treatment of overdosage.

11. *Description*. An explanation of the medication, the form in which it is administered (e.g. tablet, liquid, cream), and the concentration of active ingredients.

12. *Clinical pharmacology*. A description of how the medication is absorbed, metabolized and excreted by the body, and any known interactions that might occur if taking other medications simultaneously.

13. *Nonclinical pharmacology*. Scientific studies performed in animal models.

14. *Clinical studies*. An overview of significant clinical studies that tested the medication's intended and unintended effects on a large population of patients.

15. *References*. A list of relevant publications related to information provided in the package insert (optional).

16. *How supplied/ Storage and handling*. A description of the packaging and storage methods for each form of the medication.

17. *Patient counseling information*. A less technical, question-and-answer format of critical information regarding the medication.

Because we are focusing on the risk profiles of Premarin[®] Vaginal Cream and Osphena™, we will limit our discussion to the sections that are referenced in the boxed warnings, namely "Warnings and precautions" (Section 5), "Use in specific populations" (Section 8), and "Clinical studies" (Section 14). We will also briefly review "Adverse reactions" (Section 6). The other Sections (1-4, 7, 9-13, 15-17) are beyond the scope of this book, but they are all relevant for anyone considering the use of either Premarin[®] Vaginal Cream or Osphena™, and we encourage you to discuss them with your doctor.

Premarin® Vaginal Cream Package Insert

When you first peruse the package insert for Premarin® Vaginal Cream, you might be surprised by its sheer size [1]. At 44 pages depending on the format, it is a wealth of information, albeit mostly in medical jargon. The most important health studies on hormonal therapy to date for postmenopausal women have been the Women's Health Initiative (WHI) studies of estrogen plus progestin and estrogen alone, a research project funded by the federal government and lasting over 15 years that involved approximately 27,000 postmenopausal women to address cardiovascular disease, cancer, cognition and osteoporosis. Most of the warnings in the package insert for Premarin® Vaginal Cream are based on results from the WHI studies, and Section 14.2 is dedicated to a discussion of the WHI. It is important to note that the WHI results include a variety of substudies (i.e. smaller studies within the two main studies) intended to address specific populations and specific therapies; for example, the WHI Memory Study (WHIMS) in postmenopausal women aged 65-79 years [4, 5]. The estrogen-alone study was stopped early after an average of approximately seven years of treatment because of a significantly increased risk of stroke without any overall health benefits [2]. The estrogen plus progestin study was also stopped early after about 5.5 years of treatment due to significantly increased risks of breast cancer and cardiovascular events [3]. Recently, the latest extended follow-up findings from this trial, extending to eight years after the treatment phase ended in 2002, showed that the risk of invasive breast cancer was still significantly higher among the women treated with estrogen plus progestin compared to the placebo group [17].

Turning your attention to Section 5 of the Premarin® Vaginal Cream package insert, you will see that the warnings and precautions have been divided into 21 sub-sections so that each health issue can be distinctly addressed. If you recall, the boxed warning only highlighted four health issues (i.e. endometrial cancer, cardiovascular disorders, breast cancer, and dementia). We will address these four issues first, and then identify the remaining 17.

Section 5.3 focuses on malignant neoplasms (i.e. endometrial cancer, breast cancer, ovarian cancer), which the boxed warning referenced on two occasions. Many studies involving the use of Premarin® have occurred over the years, and this section notes that the risk of developing endometrial cancer in postmenopausal women with a uterus increases 2 to 12 times (i.e. 100% to

1100%) when taking Premarin® alone (i.e. without a progestin). The risk does not appear to be significant when the therapy is taken for less than one year, but it can climb as high as 24 times with prolonged use of five to ten years. Even more concerning, this risk can persist for up to 15 years after therapy is discontinued [18].

The results of the WHI study of estrogen plus progestin suggest that the overall risk of developing breast cancer increases 24% when Premarin® is taken in combination with a progestin [3]. However, it appears that prior use of hormone therapy is relevant. The increased risk was as high as 86% for women who reported prior use of estrogen therapies, but as low as 9% for women who reported no prior use [19].

Section 5.2 adds detail to the cardiovascular disorders (i.e. stroke, heart disease, venous thromboembolism) highlighted in the boxed warning. For women aged 50-79 years, the WHI results suggest that a statistically significant 32% increased risk of stroke exists when taking estrogen plus progestin [20]. Furthermore, estrogen-alone therapy appears to impact only women over the age of 59 when considering stroke risk. In the estrogen-alone study overall, the risk of stroke was increased by 36% with estrogen treatment compared to placebo, while no increased risk with estrogen treatment was seen among those women aged 50-59 [20]. Again citing the WHI, venous thromboembolism risk increased 36% with estrogen-alone therapy [21], and 2-fold (i.e. 100% increase) with estrogen plus progestin [22]. Venous thromboembolism includes deep vein thrombosis (blood clots in a deep vein such as in the lower leg) and pulmonary embolism (blood clots that become lodged in the lungs, blocking the blood flow through the pulmonary artery, which delivers blood from the heart to the lungs).

Section 5.4 and Section 8.5 discuss probable dementia, referencing an ancillary study of the WHI called the Women's Health Initiative Memory Study (WHIMS) that included a population of nearly 7,500 postmenopausal women aged 65-79 years (2,947 in the estrogen-alone study and 4,532 in the estrogen plus progestin study). The reported risk of developing dementia, the most common form of which was Alzheimer's disease, from estrogen alone increased 49% compared to placebo, while the risk from estrogen plus progestin increased 2-fold. When the patient populations from both studies were combined, the overall increased risk of probable dementia was 76% [4, 5]. However, no studies were conducted on women younger than 65, so the impact on younger postmenopausal women is not known.

Other warnings and precautions from Section 5 include the following adverse reactions that have been noted in postmenopausal women receiving estrogens: gallbladder disease, hypercalcemia, visual abnormalities, elevated blood pressure, hypertriglyceridemia, hepatic impairment, hypothyroidism, fluid retention, hypocalcemia, exacerbation of endometriosis, anaphylactic reaction, angioedema, hereditary angioedema. All of these conditions were observed as statistically significant during the WHI study, but they were not deemed severe enough to be mentioned in the boxed warning [1].

In addition, Section 6 identifies the following adverse reactions that have been reported by patients during post-approval use of Premarin® Vaginal Cream: abnormal uterine bleeding or spotting, dysmenorrhea (i.e. pelvic pain), increased size of uterine leiomyomata (i.e. uterine fibroids), vaginitis (i.e. inflammation of the vagina), change in cervical secretion, cystitis-like syndrome (i.e. bladder pain), application site reactions of vulvovaginal discomfort (e.g. itching, burning, rawness, irritation), precocious puberty (i.e. early hormonal changes in the body), leukorrhea (i.e. thick vaginal discharge), breast tenderness and discharge, nausea, vomiting, abdominal cramps, bloating, gallbladder disease, chloasma (i.e. large brown patches on skin and face), loss of scalp hair, hirsutism (abnormal hair growth on the face and body), rash, retinal vascular thrombosis (i.e. blockage of veins in the eye), intolerance to contact lenses, headache, migraine, dizziness, mental depression, nervousness, mood disturbances, irritability, dementia (i.e. mental incapacity), glucose intolerance, edema (i.e. excessive fluid retention), arthralgias (i.e. joint pain), leg cramps, urticaria (i.e. skin rash), exacerbation of asthma, increased triglycerides, hypersensitivity. Because these reactions were voluntarily reported from a population of indeterminate size, it is not always possible to establish a causal relationship with exposure to Premarin® Vaginal Cream or to reliably estimate the frequency of these symptoms. Therefore, these reactions should be considered a possibility without a definitive likelihood [1].

Osphena™ Package Insert

The package insert for Osphena™ is substantially smaller than the one for Premarin® Vaginal Cream [7]. At only 13 pages, you might wonder if some content is missing. The reality is that Osphena™ has far fewer warnings and adverse effects than Premarin® Vaginal Cream, and so there is less for the package insert to discuss. Section 5 of the Osphena™ package insert contains only three sub-sections of warnings and precautions, which include cardiovascular disorders, malignant neoplasms, and severe hepatic impairment. The boxed warning references only cardiovascular disorders and endometrial cancer, but we will address all three health issues here.

The cardiovascular disorders discussed in Section 5.1 are separated into three categories, all with data referenced from the same WHI studies that were used to evaluate Premarin® Vaginal Cream. Just like the Premarin® Vaginal Cream package insert, the Osphena™ package insert states that a 36% increased risk of stroke was revealed by the WHI in postmenopausal women aged 50-79 years receiving *estrogen therapy* [21]. Remember that Osphena™ is not an estrogen; it is a SERM. In the Osphena™ clinical trials with treatment up to 15 months, the incidence of thrombotic stroke—a stroke caused by a blood clot that blocks the flow of blood through a vessel in the brain—actually declined 30%, while the incidence of hemorrhagic stroke—a stroke due to bleeding; for example, a burst blood vessel in the brain—increased 1.45 per 1,000 women. In all of the Phase II and Phase III clinical trials of ospemifene, only two strokes were seen out of 1,892 women receiving ospemifene treatment, which gives an incidence of approximately 0.1% [8-13, 23, 24]. Among the 958 women receiving placebo in the various ospemifene clinical trials, one stroke was observed, which also gives an approximate 0.1% incidence [11]. Thus, the incidence of stroke seen with ospemifene treatment is virtually identical to placebo, meaning that if ospemifene does carry an increased risk of stroke, it was too small to detect in the clinical trials conducted to date. Also worth noting, the increased incidence of stroke in women participating in the clinical trials of toremifene therapy (i.e. the parent drug of Osphena™) was not statistically significant [15].

The second category of Section 5.1 discusses coronary heart disease, and again the WHI estrogen-alone study is referenced, stating that no coronary heart disease events were reported in women receiving estrogen-alone therapy [1]. In the clinical trials for Osphena™, only one heart attack was observed, and this occurred in a patient with pre-existing cardiac disease and a long history of type 2 diabetes mellitus and hypertension [12].

The third category of Section 5.1 is venous thromboembolism (i.e. blood clots). Once again the WHI estrogen-alone study is referenced, where the incidence of deep vein thrombosis increased 47% [2]. In the Osphena™ clinical trials, the incidence of deep vein thrombosis increased only 39% [7]. To understand what this 39% increase really means in terms of risk to you, the package insert specifically notes that 1.45 per thousand women (i.e. less than two women in 1,000) experienced deep vein thrombosis while on Osphena™ therapy, while 1.04 per thousand women who were in the placebo group (i.e.

not receiving Osphena™ therapy) experienced deep vein thrombosis. This yields a net increase of 0.41 events in every 1,000 women... a very small number.

Endometrial cancer risk is discussed in depth within Section 5.2 of the Osphena™ package insert. Here the FDA recognizes that Osphena™ is not a pure estrogen, but rather a SERM with tissue selective effects, meaning that it behaves like an estrogen in only some areas of the body. In the clinical trials of Osphena™, no cases of endometrial cancer were identified [8-13]. However, clinically relevant endometrial thickening (a potential precursor to endometrial health issues) increased by 3.89% (38.9 out of every 1,000 women) compared to placebo in the Osphena™ clinical trials [7]. This suggests that fewer than 4% of women might experience endometrial thickening as a result of Osphena™ therapy. If you are interested in learning more about the clinical trials of Osphena™, Chapter 4 contains detailed discussions of all of them. Section 14 of the package insert also discusses the Osphena™ clinical trials in more depth [7].

In Section 5.3, the FDA offers a single comment regarding severe hepatic impairment (i.e. liver damage), stating that women with this pre-existing condition should not use Osphena™. The reason for this warning is that Osphena™, like most drugs, is metabolized in the body by the liver. If you have liver damage, then it is possible that any compound normally metabolized by the liver could end up accumulating in other areas of the body, potentially resulting in toxic drug concentrations. Osphena™ has not been specifically studied in women with liver damage, so the FDA has simply inserted this warning as a cautionary measure [7].

Along with the warnings from Section 5, the FDA also lists other potential adverse reactions in Section 6, as identified during the clinical trials for Osphena™. They include hot flushes, also known as hot flashes (7.5% occurrence), vaginal discharge (3.8%), genital discharge (1.3%), muscle spasms (3.2%), and sweating (1.6%) [7].

Conclusion

Boxed warnings and package inserts are an effective method for educating doctors and patients about the potential health risks of medications. When reading warning labels, it is important to keep in mind that the FDA frequently chooses to err on the side of caution in favor of the patient in order to avoid any potential for surprise adverse effects. In the case of Premarin® Vaginal Cream, a long history of clinical monitoring has resulted in a comprehensive understanding of its likely adverse effects. In the case of Osphena™, specific clinical trials have demonstrated a favorable risk profile compared to Premarin® Vaginal Cream. However, without a decade or more of history on the open market, the FDA has chosen to label Osphena™ with similar long-term risks as estrogens. The reality is that Osphena™ is not an estrogen; it is a selective estrogen receptor modulator (SERM) that behaves like estrogen only in certain tissues of the body like the vagina and bone, while it opposes the effects of estrogen in other tissues such as the breast. Osphena™ is also a metabolite of toremifene, a SERM used for the treatment of metastatic breast cancer that has been on the open market for 17 years in the United States. Toremifene does not carry any of the boxed warnings that estrogens carry, and so we question why the FDA has chosen to label Osphena™ with estrogen-specific warnings. When evaluating your options for treating dyspareunia, it is important to understand which risks of a given therapy are real and which are merely assumed without actual evidence.

Table 5.7. Premarin® (conjugated estrogens) Vaginal Cream– Full Prescribing Information Contents

1.	**Indications and usage**
1.1.	Treatment of atrophic vaginitis and kraurosis vulvae
1.2.	Treatment of moderate to severe dyspareunia, a symptom of vulvar and vaginal atrophy, due to menopause
2.	**Dosage and administration**
2.1.	Treatment of moderate to severe dyspareunia, a symptom of vulvar and vaginal atrophy, due to menopause
3.	**Dosage forms and strengths**
4.	**Contraindications**
5.	**Warnings and precautions**
5.1.	Risks from systemic absorption
5.2.	Cardiovascular disorders
5.3.	Malignant neoplasms
5.4.	Probable dementia
5.5.	Gallbladder disease
5.6.	Hypercalcemia
5.7.	Visual abnormalities
5.8.	Addition of a progestin when a woman has not had a hysterectomy
5.9.	Elevated blood pressure
5.10.	Hypertriglyceridemia
5.11.	Hepatic impairment and/or past history of cholestatic jaundice
5.12.	Hypothyroidism

Table 5.7. (Continued).

5.13.	Fluid retention
5.14.	Hypocalcemia
5.15.	Exacerbation of endometriosis
5.16.	Anaphylactic reaction and angioedema
5.17.	Hereditary angioedema
5.18.	Exacerbation of other conditions
5.19.	Effects on barrier contraception
5.20.	Laboratory tests
5.21.	Drug-laboratory test interactions

6. Adverse reactions
  6.1.   Clinical trials experience
  6.2.   Postmarketing experience
7. Drug interactions
  7.1.   Metabolic interactions
8. Use in specific populations
  8.1.   Pregnancy
  8.2.   Nursing mothers
  8.3.   Pediatric use
  8.4.   Geriatric use
  8.5.   Renal impairment
  8.6.   Hepatic impairment
9. Drug Abuse and Dependence *(not included)*
10. Overdosage
11. Description
12. Clinical Pharmacology
  12.1. Mechanism of action
  12.2. Pharmacodynamics
  12.3. Pharmacokinetics
13. Nonclinical toxicology
  13.1. Carcinogenesis, mutagenesis, impairment of fertility
14. Clinical studies
  14.1. Effects on vulvar and vaginal atrophy
  14.2. Women's Health Initiative studies
  14.3. Women's Health Initiative Memory Study
15. References
16. How Supplied/ Storage and Handing
  16.1. How supplied
  16.2. Storage and handling
17. Patient counseling information
  17.1. Vaginal bleeding
  17.2. Possible serious adverse reactions with estrogen-alone therapy
  17.3. Possible less serious but common adverse reactions with estrogen-alone therapy
  17.4. Instructions for use of applicator

**Table 5.8. Osphena™ (ospemifene) Tablets – Full Prescribing
Information Contents**

1. **Indications and usage**
2. **Dosage and administration**
   2.1.   Treatment of moderate to severe dyspareunia, a symptom of vulvar and vaginal atrophy, due to menopause
3. **Dosage forms and strengths**
4. **Contraindications**
5. **Warnings and precautions**
   5.1.   Cardiovascular disorders
   5.2.   Malignant neoplasms
   5.3.   Severe hepatic impairment
6. **Adverse reactions**
   6.1.   Clinical trials experience
7. **Drug interactions**
   7.1.   Estrogens and estrogen agonist/antagonist
   7.2.   Fluconazole
   7.3.   Rifampin
   7.4.   Ketoconazole
   7.5.   Warfarin
   7.6.   Highly protein-bound drugs
   7.7.   Multiple enzyme inhibition
8. **Use in specific populations**
   8.1.   Pregnancy
   8.2.   Nursing mothers
   8.3.   Pediatric use
   8.4.   Geriatric use
   8.5.   Renal impairment
   8.6.   Hepatic impairment
9. **Drug Abuse and Dependence** *(not included)*
10. **Overdosage**
11. **Description**
12. **Clinical Pharmacology**
    12.1. Mechanism of action
    12.2. Pharmacokinetics
13. **Nonclinical toxicology**
    13.1. Carcinogenesis, mutagenesis, impairment of fertility
14. **Clinical studies**
15. **References** *(not included)*
16. **How Supplied/ Storage and handling**
    16.1. How supplied
    16.2. Storage and handling
17. **Patient counseling information**
    17.1. Hot flashes or flushes
    17.2. Vaginal bleeding

References

[1]   Premarin® (conjugated estrogens) Vaginal Cream Prescribing Information. Phildelphia, Pennsylvania: Wyeth Pharmaceuticals, Inc.; 2014.

[2]   Anderson, G. L., Limacher, M., Assaf, A. R., Bassford, T., Beresford, S. A., Black, H., et al. (2004). Effects of conjugated equine estrogen in postmenopausal women with hysterectomy: the Women's Health Initiative randomized controlled trial. *JAMA, 291(14)*, 1701-1712.

[3]   Rossouw, J. E., Anderson, G. L., Prentice, R. L., LaCroix, A. Z., Kooperberg, C., Stefanick, M. L., et al. (2002). Risks and benefits of estrogen plus progestin in healthy postmenopausal women: principal results From the Women's Health Initiative randomized controlled trial. *JAMA, 288(3)*, 321-333.

[4]   Shumaker, S. A., Legault, C., Kuller, L., Rapp, S. R., Thal, L., Lane, D. S., et al. (2004). Conjugated equine estrogens and incidence of probable dementia and mild cognitive impairment in postmenopausal women: Women's Health Initiative Memory Study. *JAMA, 291(24)*, 2947-2958.

[5]   Shumaker, S. A., Legault, C., Rapp, S. R., Thal, L., Wallace, R. B., Ockene, J. K., et al. (2003). Estrogen plus progestin and the incidence of dementia and mild cognitive impairment in postmenopausal women: the Women's Health Initiative Memory Study: a randomized controlled trial. *JAMA, 289(20)*, 2651-2662.

[6]   Stefanick, M. L. (2005). Estrogens and progestins: background and history, trends in use, and guidelines and regimens approved by the US Food and Drug Administration. *Am J Med, 118 Suppl 12B*, 64-73.

[7]   Osphena™ (ospemifene) Prescribing Information. Florham Park, New Jersey: Shionogi Inc.; 2013.

[8]   Bachmann, G. A., Komi, J. O. (2010). Ospemifene effectively treats vulvovaginal atrophy in postmenopausal women: results from a pivotal phase 3 study. *Menopause, 17(3)*, 480-486.

[9]   Goldstein, S. R., Bachmann, G. A., Koninckx, P. R., Lin, V. H., Portman, D. J., Ylikorkala, O. (2014). Ospemifene 12-month safety and efficacy in postmenopausal women with vulvar and vaginal atrophy. *Climacteric, 17(2)*, 173-182.

[10] Portman, D., Palacios, S., Nappi, R. E., Mueck, A. O. (2014). Ospemifene, a non-oestrogen selective oestrogen receptor modulator for the treatment of vaginal dryness associated with postmenopausal vulvar

and vaginal atrophy: A randomised, placebo-controlled, phase III trial. *Maturitas*, *78(2)*, 91-98.

[11] Portman, D. J., Bachmann, G. A., Simon, J. A. (2013). Ospemifene, a novel selective estrogen receptor modulator for treating dyspareunia associated with postmenopausal vulvar and vaginal atrophy. *Menopause*, *20(6)*, 623-630.

[12] Simon, J., Portman, D., Mabey, R. G., Jr. (2014). Long-term safety of ospemifene (52-week extension) in the treatment of vulvar and vaginal atrophy in hysterectomized postmenopausal women. *Maturitas*, *77(3)*, 274-281.

[13] Simon, J. A., Lin, V. H., Radovich, C., Bachmann, G. A. (2013). One-year long-term safety extension study of ospemifene for the treatment of vulvar and vaginal atrophy in postmenopausal women with a uterus. *Menopause*, *20(4)*, 418-427.

[14] Goldstein, S. R. (2013). Postmenopausal dyspareunia: has the Food and Drug Administration really helped? *Menopause*, *20(6)*, 596-597.

[15] Fareston® (toremifene citrate) Prescribing Information. Bridgewater, New Jersey: ProStrakan, Inc.; 2012.

[16] US-Food-and-Drug-Administration. PLR Requirements for Prescribing Information. U.S. Food and Drug Administration; 2006 [July 25, 2014]; Available from: http://www.fda.gov/drugs/guidancecomplianceregulatoryinformation/lawsactsandrules/ucm084159.htm.

[17] Manson, J. E., Chlebowski, R. T., Stefanick, M. L., Aragaki, A. K., Rossouw, J. E., Prentice, R. L., et al. (2013). Menopausal hormone therapy and health outcomes during the intervention and extended poststopping phases of the Women's Health Initiative randomized trials. *JAMA*, *310(13)*, 1353-1368.

[18] Grady, D., Gebretsadik, T., Kerlikowske, K., Ernster, V., Petitti, D. (1995). Hormone replacement therapy and endometrial cancer risk: a meta-analysis. *Obstet Gynecol*, *85(2)*, 304-313.

[19] Chlebowski, R. T., Hendrix, S. L., Langer, R. D., Stefanick, M. L., Gass, M., Lane, D., et al. (2003). Influence of estrogen plus progestin on breast cancer and mammography in healthy postmenopausal women: the Women's Health Initiative Randomized Trial. *JAMA*, *289(24)*, 3243-3253.

[20] Rossouw, J. E., Prentice, R. L., Manson, J. E., Wu, L., Barad, D., Barnabei, V. M., et al. (2007). Postmenopausal hormone therapy and risk of cardiovascular disease by age and years since menopause. *JAMA*, *297(13)*, 1465-1477.

risk of cardiovascular disease by age and years since menopause. *JAMA*, *297(13)*, 1465-1477.

[21]   Curb, J. D., Prentice, R. L., Bray, P. F., Langer, R. D., Van Horn, L., Barnabei, V. M., et al. (2006). Venous thrombosis and conjugated equine estrogen in women without a uterus. *Arch Intern Med*, *166(7)*, 772-780.

[22]   Cushman, M., Kuller, L. H., Prentice, R., Rodabough, R. J., Psaty, B. M., Stafford, R. S., et al. (2004). Estrogen plus progestin and risk of venous thrombosis. *JAMA*, *292(13)*, 1573-1580.

[23]   Komi, J., Lankinen, K. S., Harkonen, P., DeGregorio, M. W., Voipio, S., Kivinen, S., et al. (2005). Effects of ospemifene and raloxifene on hormonal status, lipids, genital tract, and tolerability in postmenopausal women. *Menopause*, *12(2)*, 202-209.

[24]   Rutanen, E. M., Heikkinen, J., Halonen, K., Komi, J., Lammintausta, R., Ylikorkala, O. (2003). Effects of ospemifene, a novel SERM, on hormones, genital tract, climacteric symptoms, and quality of life in postmenopausal women: a double-blind, randomized trial. *Menopause*, *10(5)*, 433-439.

Chapter 6

What Are the Effects
of Osphena™ on Bone?

Abstract

Osteoporosis (i.e. bone loss) is a chronic condition commonly seen in postmenopausal women. Low levels of estrogen due to menopause lead to an imbalance in the formation and breakdown (i.e. resorption of bone), which results in a loss of bone mineral density and weaker more porous bones that have an increased risk of fracture, especially in the hip and spine. When tamoxifen first entered use for the treatment of breast cancer in the 1970s, it was thought that because of its antiestrogenic effects, tamoxifen might cause increased bone loss and osteoporosis in postmenopausal women. However, clinical data soon began to reveal that rather than increasing bone loss, tamoxifen was having an estrogen-like effect, helping maintain bone strength and even increasing it in some cases. The closely related breast cancer drug toremifene was found to have similar effects in bone. This multifunctional nature of the selective estrogen receptor modulators (SERMs) stimulated research efforts to develop new agents that could prevent bone loss and osteoporosis more effectively than tamoxifen but with fewer side effects. These efforts culminated in the U.S. Food and Drug Administration (FDA) approval of the SERM raloxifene for the prevention and treatment of postmenopausal osteoporosis and the approval of the newest SERM bazedoxifene combined with Premarin® (conjugated estrogens) for the prevention of postmenopausal osteoporosis in 2013. As a single agent, bazedoxifene has also been approved in Europe for the treatment of postmenopausal osteoporosis in women at increased risk of fracture and in Japan for the treatment of osteoporosis in postmenopausal women. Approved by the FDA in 2013 for the treatment of painful intercourse (dyspareunia) associated with vulvar and vaginal atrophy (VVA) due to menopause, Osphena™ (ospemifene), introduced in Chapter 4, is another SERM with beneficial effects in bone, and it was studied as a potential osteoporosis drug in preclinical animal studies and early clinical trials. While additional clinical study is needed, the available data show that ospemifene poses no bone safety concerns and in fact has bone-sparing effects similar to raloxifene. Ospemifene may potentially be useful for preserving bone strength in breast cancer patients taking aromatase inhibitors, which cause bone loss and increase the risk of osteoporosis.

Introduction

Low levels of circulating estrogen in postmenopausal women lead to an imbalance in bone formation and bone breakdown (i.e. resorption), collectively known as bone turnover, which can eventually lead to weaker, porous bones and an increased risk of fracture [1]. The connection between low ovarian hormone levels and osteoporosis was first reported more than 70 years ago [2]. Osteoporosis affects approximately eight million women in the United States and is associated with an increased risk of hospitalization and death, particularly following spine and hip fractures [3, 4]. In fact, hip fractures are responsible for approximately half of all fracture-related deaths in women, and vertebral fractures are responsible for another 28% of deaths due to fracture [1]. At the age of 50, women have a 60% lifetime risk of experiencing a bone fracture due to osteoporosis, and a 16% risk of a hip fracture [5].

Postmenopausal women typically experience rapid bone loss during the first five to seven years after menopause, particularly in the spine where bone mineral density can decrease by up to 30% [6]. It is during this period that treatment can be most effective in preserving bone mass. As discussed in Chapter 3, Premarin® is very effective in preventing bone loss, but it must be taken continuously to receive any benefit. After stopping hormone therapy, postmenopausal women will experience rapid bone loss. The risk of serious side effects, however, increases with the duration of use [7, 8]. The recognition that SERMs such as tamoxifen have positive, bone-sparing effects has resulted in the development of new and safer alternatives to the use of estrogen-based therapies for the prevention of osteoporosis in postmenopausal women.

When tamoxifen became available for the treatment of breast cancer, it was thought that, because it was an antiestrogen, it might cause increased bone loss [9, 10]. It was soon discovered that instead of having a detrimental effect on bone, tamoxifen was preventing bone loss and even increasing bone mineral density in postmenopausal breast cancer patients [9]. In other words, it was acting in an estrogen-like manner in bone. The realization that tamoxifen was exerting a mixture of antiestrogenic and estrogenic effects in different tissues (i.e. it was acting like a SERM) led to the development of newer SERMs with beneficial estrogenic and antiestrogenic effects and fewer of the side effects seen with tamoxifen such as an increased risk of uterine cancer. While many of these agents failed in clinical development due to uterine safety concerns [11], raloxifene [12] and bazedoxifene, alone [13-15] and combined with conjugated estrogens [16, 17], each demonstrated beneficial effects on bone in clinical trials. As a result, raloxifene, sold under the trade name Evista® and bazedoxifene/conjugated estrogens, sold under the trade name Duavee™, received U.S. Food and Drug Administration (FDA) approval for the prevention of osteoporosis in 1997 and 2013, respectively. Raloxifene was additionally approved for the treatment of postmenopausal osteoporosis in 1999. Bazedoxifene as a single agent was approved in Europe (trade name Conbriza®) in 2009 and in Japan (trade name Viviant™) in 2010 for the treatment of osteoporosis. As a single agent drug, bazedoxifene has not yet received FDA approval.

After extensive clinical study for its effects in postmenopausal osteoporosis, breast cancer prevention and vulvar and vaginal atrophy (VVA) due to menopause, another SERM, lasofoxifene, was actually approved for the treatment of osteoporosis in Europe in 2009. However lasofoxifene, to be sold under the trade name Fablyn™, was never marketed in Europe, and as a result its marketing authorization from the European Medicines Agency expired in 2012. The clinical development of lasofoxifene, which has not been approved by the FDA, is apparently on hold due to uterine safety concerns [18], and the future of this product is uncertain.

This Chapter will discuss the bone-sparing benefits of tamoxifen, the closely related SERM toremifene, raloxifene, bazedoxifene, and the newly approved bazedoxifene/conjugated estrogens combination treatment. Included will be a discussion summarizing the known bone benefits of Osphena™ (ospemifene) and its potential for use in the prevention of osteoporosis and preserving bone strength in breast cancer patients being treated with aromatase inhibitors such as letrozole and anastrozole, which cause extremely low levels of estrogen and increase bone loss and the risk of osteoporosis [19].

The Effects of Tamoxifen and Toremifene in Bone

Although tamoxifen is not FDA approved for the treatment or prevention of postmenopausal osteoporosis, it does exert estrogen-like, bone-sparing effects in postmenopausal women. In a small two-year study conducted in 140 postmenopausal women with breast cancer, bone mineral density in the spine increased by 0.61% per year in the women taking tamoxifen compared to a 1% annual decrease in those women taking a placebo. Bone mineral density is a measure of the calcium and other minerals that make up the bone, and it is commonly measured to assess general bone health. When bone mineral density changes in the radius, which is one of the two long bones in the forearm, were assessed, decreases in the two groups of women were approximately equal [9]. Further evidence of tamoxifen's bone benefits was found in a study involving 179 healthy pre- and postmenopausal women who had participated in the Royal Marsden breast cancer prevention trial. Among the postmenopausal women taking tamoxifen, bone mineral density in the spine and hip increased by 1.17% and 1.71% per year, respectively, over the three-year period compared to slight losses in the women taking the placebo. However, among the premenopausal women, tamoxifen had the opposite effect, causing significant bone mineral density losses in the spine and hip. The premenopausal women taking tamoxifen experienced an average bone mineral density loss of 1.44% per year, while the women taking the placebo saw small annual increases [10]. This negative effect of tamoxifen on bone in premenopausal women was further supported by the results of two additional studies of women with early breast cancer, where tamoxifen treatment was associated with significant declines in bone mineral density [20, 21]. Thus, tamoxifen's activity in bone switches from estrogenic in postmenopausal women to antiestrogenic in premenopausal women.

Toremifene, a SERM closely related to tamoxifen, has also been associated with favorable bone-sparing effects. Toremifene has been shown to be as effective as tamoxifen with respect to improvement in bone mineral density in postmenopausal women with breast cancer. A study involving 121 postmenopausal breast cancer patients assigned to take either tamoxifen or toremifene daily for three years found that toremifene was equivalent to tamoxifen in preventing bone loss in the spine and femur, which is the large bone found in the thigh [22]. In a related study, this same research group evaluated the effects of toremifene compared to tamoxifen on bone mineral density in 61 postmenopausal breast cancer patients, some of whom recently discontinued hormone replacement therapy (HRT). As pointed out earlier, rapid bone loss occurs in women when they stop taking hormone replacement therapy. In this study, toremifene and tamoxifen were equally effective in reducing losses in bone mineral density among the women who had recently stopped hormone replacement therapy after their breast cancer diagnosis [23]. Further evidence that toremifene is similar to tamoxifen in preventing bone loss was found in a small study conducted in 30 postmenopausal breast cancer patients that assessed well-known indicators of bone resorption found in the urine [24]. An earlier study performed by this research group, however, found that toremifene was inferior to tamoxifen. This study found that while tamoxifen increased bone mineral density, toremifene merely prevented the normal loss associated with increasing age [25]. Furthermore, toremifene was found to be effective, but inferior to hormone replacement therapy, in preventing osteoporosis in a study involving 198 postmenopausal women aged 55 and older [26]. As mentioned earlier, one of the major metabolites of toremifene is ospemifene, and it is possible that the bone benefits observed in postmenopausal women with breast cancer taking toremifene may at least partially derive from circulating levels of ospemifene. Like tamoxifen, toremifene is not FDA approved for the prevention or treatment of postmenopausal osteoporosis.

Raloxifene for the Prevention and Treatment of Osteoporosis

Raloxifene, currently being sold under the trade name Evista®, was originally developed as a breast cancer drug, but after disappointing clinical trials results, its development for breast cancer was discontinued [27]. However, the recognition of the positive effects of SERMs on bone [28] led to the development of raloxifene as a drug for osteoporosis. In a study involving 601 healthy postmenopausal women, patients who received raloxifene treatment daily for two years experienced significant increases in bone mineral density in the spine, hip and total body compared to the women treated with a placebo, where bone mineral density in these regions decreased. Raloxifene treatment also significantly decreased overall bone turnover, which encompasses bone formation and bone resorption [12]. These positive results led to the FDA approval of raloxifene for the *prevention* of osteoporosis in postmenopausal women in 1997.

A larger clinical study known as the Multiple Outcomes of Raloxifene Evaluation (MORE) trial led to the FDA approval of raloxifene for the *treatment* of postmenopausal osteoporosis in 1999. In the MORE trial, which enrolled a total of 7,705 postmenopausal women with osteoporosis, women were assigned to take raloxifene or placebo daily for three years. Compared to women receiving the placebo, raloxifene treatment was found to significantly increase bone mineral density in the spine and femur and to reduce the risk and severity of vertebral fractures both in women with and without existing fractures at the beginning of the study. No meaningful differences were observed between raloxifene treatment and placebo with respect to non-vertebral fractures such as those of the hip, wrist and ankle [29, 30]. Significantly increased bone mineral density and decreased risk of vertebral fracture were maintained through four years of treatment with raloxifene compared to placebo [31]. During the MORE study, raloxifene treatment was not associated with an increased risk of endometrial cancer [32], which was expected as raloxifene is known to have neutral to antiestrogenic effects in the uterus.

Bazedoxifene for the Prevention and Treatment of Osteoporosis

One of the newest SERMs to be developed, bazedoxifene has been studied for both the prevention and treatment of osteoporosis in postmenopausal women. In a two-year Phase III study involving 1,434 healthy postmenopausal women at increased risk for osteoporosis, bazedoxifene was evaluated for osteoporosis prevention. The women enrolled in this study were assigned to take one of three doses of bazedoxifene (10, 20 or 40 mg), raloxifene (60 mg) or placebo daily for two years. It was necessary to include raloxifene in this study because it was a SERM already approved for the prevention of postmenopausal osteoporosis, and thus any new SERM in clinical testing for the same indication must be compared to raloxifene. Bone mineral density changes in the spine, hip and femur, as well as indicators of bone turnover in the serum, were evaluated. At all doses tested, bazedoxifene treatment comparable to raloxifene, prevented bone loss with significantly higher bone mineral density at all three skeletal sites tested, compared to women treated with the placebo. Significant decreases in serum indicators of bone turnover were also observed with bazedoxifene treatment relative to placebo [33] Assessments of breast, endometrial and ovarian safety in this study revealed no concerns [34].

To evaluate the efficacy of bazedoxifene in the treatment of osteoporosis a three-year randomized, double-blind Phase III clinical trial was conducted in

7,492 postmenopausal women with osteoporosis [15]. The patients were assigned to take bazedoxifene (20 or 40 mg), raloxifene (60 mg) or placebo daily for three years. As pointed out above, raloxifene was included in this study as an active comparator because it had already obtained FDA approval for the treatment of postmenopausal osteoporosis. The primary goal of this study was to assess the risk of new vertebral fractures, with secondary goals of evaluating non-vertebral fractures, bone mineral density and serum indicators of bone turnover. Regardless of whether patients were at low or high risk of fracture, both doses of bazedoxifene and raloxifene significantly reduced the risk of new vertebral fractures compared to the placebo. With respect to non-vertebral fractures, the incidence among women treated with bazedoxifene or raloxifene was not significantly different from placebo. Among the women with the highest risk of fracture, the 20-mg dose of bazedoxifene significantly reduced the risk of non-vertebral fractures compared to raloxifene and placebo. Although bazedoxifene significantly improved bone mineral density in the spine and hip and reduced serum levels of bone turnover indicators compared to placebo, raloxifene proved to be slightly, yet still significantly, better than bazedoxifene in this study. Both raloxifene and bazedoxifene treatment were associated with significantly higher incidences of blood clots and leg cramps [15]. In a two-year extension of this study, the results showed that bazedoxifene's bone benefits in preventing vertebral fractures and increasing bone mineral density remained significant compared to placebo through five years of treatment [14]. A second two-year extension of this study showed that the bone benefits of bazedoxifene are maintained through seven years of treatment [13]. While not statistically meaningful, the incidence of ovarian cancers remained higher in women treated with bazedoxifene compared to placebo throughout seven years of treatment [13]. Bazedoxifene is currently approved for the treatment of postmenopausal osteoporosis in Europe and Japan, where it is sold under the trade names Conbriza® and Viviant™, respectively. As of July 2014, the FDA has not approved bazedoxifene as a single agent for the treatment or prevention of osteoporosis.

Bazedoxifene/Conjugated Estrogens for the Prevention of Osteoporosis

The combination of the SERM bazedoxifene with Premarin® (conjugated estrogens) is what has been termed a tissue-selective estrogen complex. In this case, bazedoxifene protects the breast and uterine tissue in postmenopausal women from the harmful effects of estrogen, while allowing estrogen to act where it is beneficial; for example, in alleviating hot flashes. One advantage of such a combination is that there is no need for a progestin in postmenopausal women with a uterus [35]. In a series of five Phase III studies called Selective estrogen Menopause And Response to Therapy (SMART), bazedoxifene/conjugated estrogens was evaluated for its effects on the endometrium, hot flashes, vulvar and vaginal atrophy, and osteoporosis [36]. The effects of bazedoxifene/conjugated estrogens in the prevention of postmenopausal osteoporosis were evaluated in the SMART-1, SMART-4 and SMART-5 studies, summarized below.

In the SMART-1 Phase III study, which was primarily designed to assess the uterine safety of bazedoxifene in combination with conjugated estrogens, there were two osteoporosis prevention substudies: one which included healthy postmenopausal women more than five years postmenopause and one that included healthy postmenopausal women 1-5 years postmenopause [16]. The reason for separating the patients this way is that women within five years of menopause are known to experience more rapid bone loss compared to women more than five years postmenopause. A total of 3,397 subjects aged 40-75 years at increased risk of osteoporosis and with an intact uterus were enrolled and received at least one dose of medication. The women were randomly assigned to treatment with one of three doses of bazedoxifene (10, 20 or 40 mg) in combination with either 0.625 or 0.45 mg conjugated estrogens, raloxifene 60 mg or placebo daily for two years. Bone mineral density changes in the spine and hip were assessed in both substudies and serum indicators of bone turnover were assessed in the women five or fewer years postmenopause. In both substudies, bone mineral density in the spine and hip increased significantly with all doses of bazedoxifene/conjugated estrogens compared to the placebo. Among the women who were within five years of postmenopause, most of the bazedoxifene and conjugated estrogen combinations increased bone mineral density significantly more than raloxifene as well. For serum indicators of bone turnover, all combinations of bazedoxifene and conjugated estrogens in both substudies resulted in significant decreases compared to placebo and when compared to raloxifene for most of the bazedoxifene combinations. This indicates that bazedoxifene/conjugated estrogens effectively increased bone mineral density and decreased bone turnover in postmenopausal women at increased risk of osteoporosis, and that bazedoxifene in combination with conjugated estrogens was generally more effective than raloxifene [16].

These positive effects of bazedoxifene combined with conjugated estrogens in the prevention of osteoporosis were reinforced by the results of the SMART-4 and SMART-5 studies, which were specifically designed to assess the effects of this combination on bone mineral density in postmenopausal women with an intact uterus. The SMART-4 study was a one-year Phase III trial of bazedoxifene 20 mg combined with 0.45 or 0.625 mg conjugated estrogens compared to placebo and standard estrogen/progestin hormone replacement therapy (0.45 mg conjugated estrogens with 1.5 mg medroxyprogesterone acetate) taken daily in 1,083 generally healthy postmenopausal women aged 40-65 years. After one year of treatment, both bazedoxifene and conjugated estrogen combinations significantly increased bone mineral density in the spine and hip compared to placebo [37]. The SMART-5 study had a similar design to SMART-4 but included a 20-mg bazedoxifene alone group. A total of 1,843 generally healthy postmenopausal women aged 40-65 years seeking treatment for menopausal symptoms were enrolled in the SMART-5 study. After daily treatments for one year, the women receiving the combinations of bazedoxifene and conjugated estrogens and bazedoxifene alone showed significantly increased bone mineral density in the spine and hip compared to women taking the placebo, who showed decreases. Women taking hormone replacement therapy showed greater increases in spinal bone mineral density compared to bazedoxifene/conjugated estrogens. Serum indicators of bone turnover were also assessed in the SMART-5 study, and the women treated with the combinations of bazedoxifene and conjugated estrogens showed significant decreases compared to placebo and to bazedoxifene alone [17]. Overall, bazedoxifene/conjugated estrogens was found to have an acceptable endometrial safety profile, although pooled safety data from all five SMART trials showed that the incidence of endometrial polyps and overall endometrium-related side effects were higher following treatment with bazedoxifene/conjugated estrogens compared to placebo [36]. In the SMART-5 study, the incidence of endometrial polyps was significantly higher with the combination of bazedoxifene 20 mg and conjugated estrogens 0.45 mg, the formulation that has been FDA approved, when compared to placebo [17].

The combination of bazedoxifene (20 mg) and conjugated estrogens (0.45 mg), currently being marketed under the trade name Duavee™, was approved by the FDA in October 2013 for the prevention of postmenopausal osteoporosis and for the treatment of moderate to severe vasomotor symptoms due to menopause. As mentioned in the Conclusion to Chapter 3, bazedoxifene (20 mg) combined with conjugated estrogens (0.45 and 0.625 mg) was also studied for the treatment of postmenopausal vulvar and vaginal atrophy. In the SMART-3 study, the combination containing 0.45 mg conjugated estrogens proved to be ineffective compared to 0.625 mg conjugated estrogens, an indication that the vulvar and vaginal atrophy benefits are likely due to the estrogen component. However, while the combination of bazedoxifene 20 mg and 0.625 mg conjugated estrogens was effective overall in treating vulvar and vaginal atrophy, it did not significantly improve the specific most bothersome symptom of dyspareunia in the SMART-3 study, and it was associated with a significantly increased incidence of vaginitis [38]. The FDA declined to approve the formulation of Duavee™ containing 20 mg of bazedoxifene and 0.625 mg conjugated estrogens for the treatment of vulvar and vaginal atrophy due to menopause, which was the only formulation for which the manufacturer sought approval.

Potential of Ospemifene for the Prevention and Treatment of Osteoporosis

Compared to raloxifene, bazedoxifene and the combination of bazedoxifene and conjugated estrogens, ospemifene has not been extensively studied for its effects in the treatment and prevention of postmenopausal osteoporosis. However, this was one of the originally targeted indications based on preclinical data, and results from two Phase II clinical trials showed that ospemifene may prove to be useful in the management of osteoporosis in postmenopausal women. The first Phase II study was a randomized, double-blind, placebo-controlled trial conducted in 159 healthy postmenopausal women. Subjects were randomized to receive one of three doses of ospemifene (30, 60 or 90 mg) or placebo daily for 12 weeks. Urinary indicators of bone resorption and serum indicators of bone formation were assessed at baseline, after 12 weeks of treatment, and then 2-4 weeks after cessation of treatment. Significant decreases in indicators of bone resorption were observed at all ospemifene dose levels compared to placebo, and the effect of ospemifene increased with dose. At the two higher doses, serum indicators of bone formation significantly decreased in response to dose compared to the placebo. When assessed 2-4 weeks after the end of treatment, all indicators of bone turnover showed clear increases. This study demonstrated that ospemifene effectively reduced bone turnover in postmenopausal women [39].

The second Phase II study examined the effects of ospemifene compared to raloxifene on the same serum and urinary indicators of bone turnover evaluated in the first study. A total of 118 healthy postmenopausal women were assigned to one of three doses of ospemifene (30, 60 or 90 mg) or raloxifene (60 mg) daily for 12 weeks. At the time this study was conducted, raloxifene had already been FDA approved for the prevention and treatment of osteoporosis, and it was thus included as an active comparator. The results showed that all doses of ospemifene and raloxifene effectively reduced urinary and serum levels of bone turnover indicators, and that the effects of ospemifene were comparable to raloxifene [40]. While both of these Phase II studies showed that ospemifene was very effective in reducing bone turnover compared to a placebo and was comparable to raloxifene, long-term studies that include bone mineral density and fracture assessments are still needed to fully assess the potential of ospemifene to treat and/or prevent osteoporosis in postmenopausal women. At the very least, these studies demonstrate that ospemifene poses no bone safety concerns in healthy postmenopausal women.

There is also an abundance of preclinical animal data demonstrating the potential utility of ospemifene in osteoporosis. Using the female rat model of postmenopausal osteoporosis, ospemifene has been extensively studied for its effects in preventing bone loss. In this rat model, the ovaries are removed to simulate the loss of estrogen seen during menopause. This results in rapid bone loss in untreated animals. Using this rat model, ospemifene was administered daily for four weeks at a low and high dose. Control rats that received no active drug experienced significant bone loss while the higher dose of ospemifene preserved bone strength and volume in the spine and femur. The higher dose of ospemifene also significantly reduced indicators of bone turnover compared to the control animals. When estrogen and ospemifene were combined in this study, no meaningful differences were observed compared to estrogen alone, indicating that ospemifene does not oppose the action of estrogen in the bone [41]. A similarly designed study showed that ospemifene was similar to raloxifene in preventing increases in indicators of bone turnover as a result of menopause [41, 42]. To determine whether ospemifene's bone-sparing effects are maintained long-term, female rats were treated daily with ospemifene for one year. Just as seen in the four-week studies, ospemifene significantly prevented menopause-induced losses in bone strength and density compared to untreated rats [42]. The overall results of these rat osteoporosis studies coupled with the Phase II clinical data supports the hypothesis that ospemifene has beneficial bone effects, similar to raloxifene, and may potentially be useful in the treatment or prevention of osteoporosis in postmenopausal women. A more detailed discussion of the effects of ospemifene in bone in preclinical animal studies can be found in Chapter 4.

Conclusion

One the most frequently asked questions about ospemifene among clinicians since the drug was approved in 2013 has been "What are the effects of ospemifene in the bone?" The SERMs raloxifene and now bazedoxifene, both alone and in combination with conjugated estrogens, have established roles in the treatment and/or prevention of postmenopausal osteoporosis. As a drug class, the SERMs are known for their positive, estrogen-like effects in bone, and ospemifene is no exception. Both tamoxifen and toremifene, currently used in breast cancer treatment, have been shown to have similar, positive effects in bone in postmenopausal women with breast cancer, and ospemifene is in the same chemical family (i.e. triphenylethylenes) as tamoxifen and toremifene. Ospemifene is, in fact, one of the major metabolites of toremifene and may contribute to the overall beneficial effects of toremifene in bone. Due to the focus on vulvar and vaginal atrophy treatment during Phase III clinical development, ospemifene was not extensively evaluated for its effects in osteoporosis as were raloxifene, bazedoxifene and bazedoxifene/conjugated estrogens; however, preclinical animal studies have shown that ospemifene effectively prevents bone loss due to menopause and that it reduces serum and urinary indicators of bone turnover in a manner similar to raloxifene, a SERM already FDA approved for the treatment and prevention of osteoporosis in postmenopausal women. In agreement with preclinical studies, two Phase II clinical studies have also found that ospemifene effectively reduces bone turnover and that it acts in a manner similar to raloxifene in postmenopausal women. It is thus apparent, based on the available scientific evidence, that ospemifene does not present any bone safety concerns, and that it is very likely instead to have beneficial effects similar to the other approved SERMs.

Additional clinical studies evaluating the effects of ospemifene on bone mineral density and bone fractures in the spine and hip in postmenopausal women at increased risk of osteoporosis and postmenopausal women with osteoporosis are needed to establish the efficacy of ospemifene in the prevention and treatment of osteoporosis. In our opinion, ospemifene will prove to be safe for use in postmenopausal breast cancer patients, who are at an increased risk of bone loss due to the use of aromatase inhibitors, which inhibit the production of estrogen in the body, and for the treatment of vulvar and vaginal atrophy in healthy postmenopausal women who are at an increased risk of developing osteoporosis. Chapter 7 will explore the effects of ospemifene and the other approved SERMs in the breast and in breast cancer.

References

[1] Reginster, J. Y., Neuprez, A., Beaudart, C., Lecart, M. P., Sarlet, N., Bernard, D., et al. (2014). Antiresorptive drugs beyond bisphosphonates and selective oestrogen receptor modulators for the management of postmenopausal osteoporosis. *Drugs Aging, 31(6)*, 413-424.

[2] Albright, F., Smith, P. H., Richardson, A. M. (1941). Postmenopausal osteoporosis: its clinical features. *JAMA, 116(22)*, 2465-2474.

[3] Cheng, H., Gary, L. C., Curtis, J. R., Saag, K. G., Kilgore, M. L., Morrisey, M. A., et al. (2009). Estimated prevalence and patterns of presumed osteoporosis among older Americans based on Medicare data. *Osteoporos Int, 20(9)*, 1507-1515.

[4] de Waure, C., Specchia, M. L., Cadeddu, C., Capizzi, S., Capri, S., Di Pietro, M. L., et al. (2014). The prevention of postmenopausal osteoporotic fractures: results of the Health Technology Assessment of a new antiosteoporotic drug. *Biomed Res Int, 2014*, 975927.

[5] Davis, S. R., Dinatale, I., Rivera-Woll, L., Davison, S. (2005). Postmenopausal hormone therapy: from monkey glands to transdermal patches. *J Endocrinol, 185(2)*, 207-222.

[6] Shifren, J. L., Schiff, I. (2010). Role of hormone therapy in the management of menopause. *Obstet Gynecol, 115(4)*, 839-855.

[7] Heiss, G., Wallace, R., Anderson, G. L., Aragaki, A., Beresford, S. A., Brzyski, R., et al. (2008). Health risks and benefits 3 years after stopping randomized treatment with estrogen and progestin. *JAMA, 299(9)*, 1036-1045.

[8] LaCroix, A. Z., Chlebowski, R. T., Manson, J. E., Aragaki, A. K., Johnson, K. C., Martin, L., et al. (2011). Health outcomes after stopping conjugated equine estrogens among postmenopausal women with prior hysterectomy: a randomized controlled trial. *JAMA, 305(13)*, 1305-1314.

[9] Love, R. R., Mazess, R. B., Barden, H. S., Epstein, S., Newcomb, P. A., Jordan, V. C., et al. (1992). Effects of tamoxifen on bone mineral density

in postmenopausal women with breast cancer. *N Engl J Med*, *326(13)*, 852-856.

[10] Powles, T. J., Hickish, T., Kanis, J. A., Tidy, A., Ashley, S. (1996). Effect of tamoxifen on bone mineral density measured by dual-energy x-ray absorptiometry in healthy premenopausal and postmenopausal women. *J Clin Oncol*, *14(1)*, 78-84.

[11] Pinkerton, J. V., Goldstein, S. R. (2010). Endometrial safety: a key hurdle for selective estrogen receptor modulators in development. *Menopause*, *17(3)*, 642-653.

[12] Delmas, P. D., Bjarnason, N. H., Mitlak, B. H., Ravoux, A. C., Shah, A. S., Huster, W. J., et al. (1997). Effects of raloxifene on bone mineral density, serum cholesterol concentrations, and uterine endometrium in postmenopausal women. *N Engl J Med*, *337(23)*, 1641-1647.

[13] Palacios, S., de Villiers, T. J., Nardone Fde, C., Levine, A. B., Williams, R., Hines, T., et al. (2013). Assessment of the safety of long-term bazedoxifene treatment on the reproductive tract in postmenopausal women with osteoporosis: results of a 7-year, randomized, placebo-controlled, phase 3 study. *Maturitas*, *76(1)*, 81-87.

[14] Silverman, S. L., Chines, A. A., Kendler, D. L., Kung, A. W., Teglbjaerg, C. S., Felsenberg, D., et al. (2012). Sustained efficacy and safety of bazedoxifene in preventing fractures in postmenopausal women with osteoporosis: results of a 5-year, randomized, placebo-controlled study. *Osteoporos Int*, *23(1)*, 351-363.

[15] Silverman, S. L., Christiansen, C., Genant, H. K., Vukicevic, S., Zanchetta, J. R., de Villiers, T. J., et al. (2008). Efficacy of bazedoxifene in reducing new vertebral fracture risk in postmenopausal women with osteoporosis: results from a 3-year, randomized, placebo-, and active-controlled clinical trial. *J Bone Miner Res*, *23(12)*, 1923-1934.

[16] Lindsay, R., Gallagher, J. C., Kagan, R., Pickar, J. H., Constantine, G. (2009). Efficacy of tissue-selective estrogen complex of bazedoxifene/conjugated estrogens for osteoporosis prevention in at-risk postmenopausal women. *Fertil Steril*, *92(3)*, 1045-1052.

[17] Pinkerton, J. V., Harvey, J. A., Lindsay, R., Pan, K., Chines, A. A., Mirkin, S., et al. (2014). Effects of bazedoxifene/conjugated estrogens on the endometrium and bone: a randomized trial. *J Clin Endocrinol Metab*, *99(2)*, E189-198.

[18] Pinkerton, J. V., Thomas, S. (2014). Use of SERMs for treatment in postmenopausal women. *J Steroid Biochem Mol Biol*, *142*, 142-154.

[19] Hadji, P. (2009). Aromatase inhibitor-associated bone loss in breast cancer patients is distinct from postmenopausal osteoporosis. *Crit Rev Oncol Hematol, 69(1)*, 73-82.

[20] Sverrisdottir, A., Fornander, T., Jacobsson, H., von Schoultz, E., Rutqvist, L. E. (2004). Bone mineral density among premenopausal women with early breast cancer in a randomized trial of adjuvant endocrine therapy. *J Clin Oncol, 22(18)*, 3694-3699.

[21] Vehmanen, L., Elomaa, I., Blomqvist, C., Saarto, T. (2006). Tamoxifen treatment after adjuvant chemotherapy has opposite effects on bone mineral density in premenopausal patients depending on menstrual status. *J Clin Oncol, 24(4)*, 675-680.

[22] Saarto, T., Blomqvist, C., Valimaki, M., Makela, P., Sarna, S., Elomaa, I. (1997). Clodronate improves bone mineral density in post-menopausal breast cancer patients treated with adjuvant antioestrogens. *Br J Cancer, 75(4)*, 602-605.

[23] Saarto, T., Vehmanen, L., Elomaa, I., Valimaki, M., Makela, P., Blomqvist, C. (2001). The effect of clodronate and antioestrogens on bone loss associated with oestrogen withdrawal in postmenopausal women with breast cancer. *Br J Cancer, 84(8)*, 1047-1051.

[24] Marttunen, M. B., Hietanen, P., Titinen, A., Roth, H. J., Viinikka, L., Ylikorkala, O. (1999). Effects of tamoxifen and toremifene on urinary excretion of pyridinoline and deoxypyridinoline and bone density in postmenopausal patients with breast cancer. *Calcif Tissue Int, 65(5)*, 365-368.

[25] Marttunen, M. B., Hietanen, P., Tiitinen, A., Ylikorkala, O. (1998). Comparison of effects of tamoxifen and toremifene on bone biochemistry and bone mineral density in postmenopausal breast cancer patients. *J Clin Endocrinol Metab, 83(4)*, 1158-1162.

[26] Harvey, H. A., Kimura, M., Hajba, A. (2006). Toremifene: an evaluation of its safety profile. *Breast, 15(2)*, 142-157.

[27] Jordan, V. C. (2003). Antiestrogens and selective estrogen receptor modulators as multifunctional medicines. 1. Receptor interactions. *J Med Chem, 46(6)*, 883-908.

[28] Jordan, V. C., Phelps, E., Lindgren, J. U. (1987). Effects of anti-estrogens on bone in castrated and intact female rats. *Breast Cancer Res Treat, 10(1)*, 31-35.

[29] Ettinger, B., Black, D. M., Mitlak, B. H., Knickerbocker, R. K., Nickelsen, T., Genant, H. K., et al. (1999). Reduction of vertebral fracture risk in postmenopausal women with osteoporosis treated with

raloxifene: results from a 3-year randomized clinical trial. Multiple Outcomes of Raloxifene Evaluation (MORE) Investigators. *JAMA*, *282(7)*, 637-645.

[30]   Siris, E., Adachi, J. D., Lu, Y., Fuerst, T., Crans, G. G., Wong, M., et al. (2002). Effects of raloxifene on fracture severity in postmenopausal women with osteoporosis: results from the MORE study. Multiple Outcomes of Raloxifene Evaluation. *Osteoporos Int*, *13(11)*, 907-913.

[31]   Delmas, P. D., Ensrud, K. E., Adachi, J. D., Harper, K. D., Sarkar, S., Gennari, C., et al. (2002). Efficacy of raloxifene on vertebral fracture risk reduction in postmenopausal women with osteoporosis: four-year results from a randomized clinical trial. *J Clin Endocrinol Metab*, *87(8)*, 3609-3617.

[32]   Grady, D., Ettinger, B., Moscarelli, E., Plouffe, L., Jr., Sarkar, S., Ciaccia, A., et al. (2004). Safety and adverse effects associated with raloxifene: multiple outcomes of raloxifene evaluation. *Obstet Gynecol*, *104(4)*, 837-844.

[33]   Miller, P. D., Chines, A. A., Christiansen, C., Hoeck, H. C., Kendler, D. L., Lewiecki, E. M., et al. (2008). Effects of bazedoxifene on BMD and bone turnover in postmenopausal women: 2-yr results of a randomized, double-blind, placebo-, and active-controlled study. *J Bone Miner Res*, *23(4)*, 525-535.

[34]   Pinkerton, J. V., Archer, D. F., Utian, W. H., Menegoci, J. C., Levine, A. B., Chines, A. A., et al. (2009). Bazedoxifene effects on the reproductive tract in postmenopausal women at risk for osteoporosis. *Menopause*, *16(6)*, 1102-1108.

[35]   Mirkin, S., Komm, B. S. (2013). Tissue-selective estrogen complexes for postmenopausal women. *Maturitas*, *76(3)*, 213-220.

[36]   Komm, B. S., Mirkin, S., Jenkins, S. N. (2014). Development of conjugated estrogens/bazedoxifene, the first tissue selective estrogen complex (TSEC) for management of menopausal hot flashes and postmenopausal bone loss. *Steroids*;10.1016/j.steroids.2014.06.004.

[37]   Mirkin, S., Komm, B. S., Pan, K., Chines, A. A. (2013). Effects of bazedoxifene/conjugated estrogens on endometrial safety and bone in postmenopausal women. *Climacteric*, *16(3)*, 338-346.

[38]   Kagan, R., Williams, R. S., Pan, K., Mirkin, S., Pickar, J. H. (2010). A randomized, placebo- and active-controlled trial of bazedoxifene/conjugated estrogens for treatment of moderate to severe vulvar/vaginal atrophy in postmenopausal women. *Menopause*, *17(2)*, 281-289.

[39] Komi, J., Heikkinen, J., Rutanen, E. M., Halonen, K., Lammintausta, R., Ylikorkala, O. (2004). Effects of ospemifene, a novel SERM, on biochemical markers of bone turnover in healthy postmenopausal women. *Gynecol Endocrinol, 18(3)*, 152-158.

[40] Komi, J., Lankinen, K. S., DeGregorio, M., Heikkinen, J., Saarikoski, S., Tuppurainen, M., et al. (2006). Effects of ospemifene and raloxifene on biochemical markers of bone turnover in postmenopausal women. *J Bone Miner Metab, 24(4)*, 314-318.

[41] Qu, Q., Zheng, H., Dahllund, J., Laine, A., Cockcroft, N., Peng, Z., et al. (2000). Selective estrogenic effects of a novel triphenylethylene compound, FC1271a, on bone, cholesterol level, and reproductive tissues in intact and ovariectomized rats. *Endocrinology, 141(2)*, 809-820.

[42] Kangas, L., Harkonen, P., Vaananen, K., Peng, Z. (2014). Effects of the selective estrogen receptor modulator ospemifene on bone in rats. *Horm Metab Res, 46(1)*, 27-35.

Chapter 7

What Are the Effects of Osphena™ in the Breast?

Abstract

After skin cancer, breast cancer is the most common form of cancer in women, with approximately 233,000 new cases and 40,000 deaths expected in the United States in 2014. The recognition that many breast cancers are dependent on estrogen for growth allowed for the development of agents that target the estrogen receptor. One such class of agents, known as selective estrogen receptor modulators (SERMs), includes tamoxifen, approved for the treatment and prevention of breast cancer; toremifene, approved for metastatic breast cancer treatment; raloxifene, approved for the prevention and treatment of postmenopausal osteoporosis and breast cancer prevention; and ospemifene, which is currently approved for the treatment of dyspareunia associated with vulvar and vaginal atrophy (VVA) due to menopause. While vulvar and vaginal atrophy is a common postmenopausal condition, it is compounded in women with breast cancer due to early menopause brought on by chemotherapy or the use of aromatase inhibitors, which are drugs that block the production of estrogen, resulting in extremely low levels of circulating estrogen. Ospemifene, which is closely related to tamoxifen and toremifene, was extensively studied in animal models to assess its potential as a breast cancer treatment and preventive agent. The results of these studies strongly suggested that ospemifene, like the other similar SERMs, acts as an antiestrogen in the breast and that its efficacy in preventing breast cancer was equivalent to that of tamoxifen. Because the focus of Phase III development was on vulvar and vaginal atrophy rather than breast cancer, the effects of ospemifene in the breast were not specifically examined. As a result, the U.S. Food and Drug Administration (FDA) required that ospemifene's label include a warning against the use of this agent in women with breast cancer or who are at a high risk of developing breast cancer, similar to conjugated equine estrogens. This was done purely on a precautionary basis and not due to any existing data suggesting that ospemifene may be harmful in this patient population. There are currently no data showing that ospemifene poses any breast-related risks. Breast cancer patients, who are unable to use estrogen-based products to alleviate their vulvar and vaginal atrophy symptoms, could benefit from the use of ospemifene, and thus future clinical studies of ospemifene in breast cancer are needed.

Introduction

Despite our ever increasing knowledge base regarding the nature of breast cancer and our best efforts in continuing to develop new and effective treatment strategies, breast cancer is still expected to claim the lives of about 40,000 women in the United States in 2014, making it the second leading cause of cancer-related deaths after lung cancer [1]. The recognition that many breast cancers are dependent on estrogen for growth made the estrogen receptor a target for treatment with a novel class of agents known as selective estrogen receptor modulators (SERMs). Perhaps the best known of these compounds is the first clinically useful SERM, tamoxifen, which has been used in the treatment of breast cancer in the United States since 1977. After the results of the Breast Cancer Prevention Trial were announced in 1998 [2], tamoxifen received additional U.S. Food and Drug Administration (FDA) approval for reducing the risk of breast cancer in women at high risk for developing the disease, making it the first drug to be approved for this indication.

Other FDA-approved SERMs that have proven to be effective in the treatment or prevention of breast cancer include toremifene, sold under the trade name Fareston®, and raloxifene, sold under the trade name Evista®. Toremifene, which is closely related to tamoxifen, differing by only a single chlorine atom, was approved by the FDA in 1997 for the treatment of metastatic breast cancer (i.e. cancer that has spread to other parts of the body), where a number of clinical trials have demonstrated it to be as effective as tamoxifen [3-7]. Raloxifene is currently FDA approved for the treatment and prevention of postmenopausal osteoporosis (see Chapter 6), but it was originally developed for use in breast cancer treatment in the 1980s [8]. Following announcement of the results from the Study of Tamoxifen and Raloxifene (STAR), which showed that raloxifene was as effective as tamoxifen in preventing invasive breast cancer [9], raloxifene received additional FDA approval for the prevention of invasive breast cancer in postmenopausal women at high risk.

Ospemifene (Osphena™) is a SERM from the same chemical class as tamoxifen and toremifene and is currently FDA approved for the treatment of dyspareunia associated with vulvar and vaginal atrophy (VVA) due to menopause. Ospemifene is in fact one of the main metabolites of toremifene, meaning that women currently taking toremifene for breast cancer have circulating levels of ospemifene in their bodies [10, 11]. While ospemifene was not specifically studied for its effects in breast cancer in clinical trials, numerous animal studies have shown that ospemifene acts as an antiestrogen in breast cancer, similar to tamoxifen, toremifene and raloxifene. These studies showed that ospemifene is as effective as tamoxifen in preventing and treating breast cancer [12-16].

One of the most frequently asked questions since the approval of ospemifene for dyspareunia has been, "What are its effects in the breast?" This question is particularly relevant for breast cancer patients because they suffer from vulvar and vaginal atrophy as a result of chemotherapy, which can cause early menopause, and the use of aromatase inhibitors, which reduce estrogen to extremely low levels. Breast cancer patients are unable to use estrogen-based products for the treatment of their symptoms due to estrogen-related risks, and thus they could greatly benefit from ospemifene. Because there is insufficient clinical data regarding the effects of ospemifene in the breast, the FDA has required the labeling to include a warning against the use of ospemifene in women with known or suspected breast cancer or who are at high risk of breast cancer. Future clinical trials addressing this issue, if positive, could potentially make a very effective treatment for vulvar and vaginal atrophy available to a currently underserved patient population.

This Chapter will summarize the known effects of tamoxifen, toremifene and raloxifene in breast cancer and give an overview of the effects of ospemifene in various preclinical animal models of breast cancer. Included will be a discussion on the frequency and severity of vulvar and vaginal atrophy symptoms in breast cancer patients.

Breast Cancer and Vulvar and Vaginal Atrophy

While many women experience symptoms of vulvar and vaginal atrophy such as vaginal dryness and painful sexual intercourse (dyspareunia) as they normally progress through the menopausal transition, these sexual problems can become more frequent and bothersome among breast cancer survivors due to the effects of chemotherapy [17-19] and adjuvant hormonal treatments such as aromatase inhibitors, e.g. anastrozole and letrozole [20-24]. In breast cancer patients, an adjuvant treatment is a therapy used following a primary treatment, usually surgery to remove the tumor, to prevent a recurrence of the disease. Among younger, premenopausal women being treated for breast cancer, the harsh effects of chemotherapy and removal of the ovaries (oophorectomy) result in the early onset of menopause, and the associated symptoms of vulvar and vaginal atrophy can be particularly distressing for these patients [19, 25, 26]. More than a quarter of all newly diagnosed breast cancer patients are aged 50 years or younger [18, 19]. The stress and worry over having breast cancer coupled with sexual problems as a result of vulvar and vaginal atrophy can lead to feelings of sexual inadequacy, loss of interest in sex, and depression in breast cancer patients, which can in turn exacerbate their vulvar and vaginal atrophy symptoms and significantly impact their overall quality of life [18, 19, 27-29]. Addressing these sexual problems in breast cancer patients has become of topic of concern [30] as more and more women are now surviving breast cancer. According to the American Cancer Society, there were estimated to be about 2.8 million breast cancer survivors in the United States as of early 2014.

Chemotherapy for breast cancer can lead to either temporary or permanent ovarian failure depending on the age of the patient, with younger patients having a greater chance of recovering ovarian function, as well as the type of chemotherapy [26, 31]. For example, female breast cancer patients aged at least 40 years treated with the chemotherapy regimen containing the drugs cyclophosphamide, melphalan and 5-fluorouracil have a greater than 80% risk of permanent ovarian failure. The same chemotherapy regimen in breast cancer patients under 30 years of age has a much lower risk of permanent ovarian failure [26]. However, even younger breast cancer patients in whom normal ovarian function resumes will experience an earlier than expected menopause due to the predictable toxic effects of chemotherapy on the ovaries [19, 32]. The resulting sudden loss of estrogen brings about abrupt symptoms of menopause, which can be particularly distressing for younger patients [25] Breast cancer patients taking aromatase inhibitors such as anastrozole and letrozole, which inhibit almost all production of estrogen in the body resulting in extremely low levels of circulating hormone, experience symptoms of vulvar and vaginal atrophy to a greater degree compared to breast cancer patients not using such therapies [20, 22]. Women taking tamoxifen can also experience increased symptoms of vulvar and vaginal atrophy, particularly dyspareunia [20]. Because of the breast cancer risks associated with estrogen-based menopausal therapy, vulvar and vaginal atrophy treatment options for women with estrogen-dependent cancers are somewhat limited. Breast cancer patients that fail to get adequate symptom relief from non-hormonal moisturizers and lubricants can discuss the use of short-course, low-dose vaginal estrogen with their doctors [33]. For women who had non-hormone-dependent breast cancers, their vulvar and vaginal atrophy symptoms can be managed similar to women without a history of breast cancer [33]. Currently, ospemifene (Osphena™) is not indicated for use in women with a history of breast cancer, but it could prove to be a valuable treatment option for breast cancer survivors suffering from vulvar and vaginal atrophy who are unable to use estrogen-based therapies and for those women whose symptoms are being exacerbated by the use of aromatase inhibitors. Future clinical trials of ospemifene in breast cancer will need to be conducted to demonstrate the safety of ospemifene in these patients.

Tamoxifen for the Treatment of Breast Cancer

Research into new contraceptive agents back in the 1950s and 1960s resulted in the development of the first clinically useful SERM, tamoxifen [8]. Ironically, rather than acting as a contraceptive, tamoxifen was found to actually induce ovulation [34], which eventually led to the approval of tamoxifen for this indication. Tamoxifen was later developed as a treatment for breast cancer due to its antiestrogenic effects in this tissue, and it is now approved for the treatment of all stages of breast cancer and for reducing the risk of breast cancer in postmenopausal women at high risk of developing the disease [35]. Tamoxifen has been in use as first-line treatment for postmenopausal breast cancer patients since 1977.

In the treatment of breast cancer, tamoxifen was first used in patients with advanced, metastatic disease, meaning that the cancer had already spread to other parts of the body. Metastatic breast cancer patients who respond best to tamoxifen are those who experience a disease-free interval of at least two years after surgery and have cancers expressing both estrogen and progesterone receptors. Overall, approximately 50% of women with metastatic breast cancer that expresses the estrogen receptor benefit from tamoxifen treatment, compared to only 5% of patients whose cancer does not have estrogen receptors [36]. Among the half of patients with metastatic disease who respond to tamoxifen, approximately 60% showed tumor regression for an average of 12 months, while the remaining 40% had stable disease for six months, meaning that their cancer did not get any worse but did not get any better either [37]. A woman's menopausal status and the expression of estrogen and progesterone receptors in her cancer have an important impact on the effectiveness of tamoxifen treatment. The presence of the progesterone receptor is an indicator of estrogen activity, and the estrogen receptor is the principal target of tamoxifen, which antagonizes (inhibits) the activity of estrogen. Among premenopausal women with estrogen receptor-positive metastatic breast cancer, the overall response rate to tamoxifen is only approximately 24%. In postmenopausal women whose cancer expresses high levels of estrogen and progesterone receptors, the tamoxifen response rate is about 86%. The response rate is lower but still clinically significant in metastatic breast cancer patients whose tumors are positive for estrogen receptor expression but negative for the progesterone receptor. For women with estrogen receptor-negative metastatic breast cancer, the response rate to tamoxifen is only 5-10% [36].

Tamoxifen has also proven to be a valuable adjuvant treatment for preventing the recurrence of breast cancer. Adjuvant therapies for breast cancer are used to prevent a second occurrence following an initial treatment, which usually includes surgery to remove the primary tumor. When data from 55 different clinical studies begun prior to 1990 and involving a total of more than 37,000 women with operable breast cancer was combined and analyzed, tamoxifen was found to significantly reduce breast cancer recurrence and deaths after 10 years of follow-up. Compared to a placebo, tamoxifen reduced the annual incidence of breast cancer recurrence and deaths by 26% and 14%, respectively, when all patients were included in the analysis. These benefits were far greater among the women who took tamoxifen for five years and in the patients whose tumors were positive for estrogen receptor expression [38]. Five years of adjuvant tamoxifen treatment for breast cancer has been the standard of care for many years, with the most recent analysis showing that disease recurrence in women with estrogen receptor-positive breast cancer was reduced by 47% during the five years of tamoxifen treatment and 32% during the five-year period after treatment was stopped compared to women who received no tamoxifen treatment. No meaningful additional reduction was seen over the ensuing five-year period. Deaths due to breast cancer were reduced by about one-third over the total 15-year period [39]. Recently published data from the Adjuvant Tamoxifen: Longer Against Shorter (ATLAS) trial, which involved nearly 7,000 women with early stage estrogen receptor-positive breast cancer, revealed that giving tamoxifen for 10 years significantly reduced disease recurrence and death due to breast cancer compared to women who received five years of treatment [40]. Because an additional five years of tamoxifen treatment also increases the risks of endometrial cancers and other potentially serious side effects, additional study will be needed to verify these results.

Tamoxifen for Breast Cancer Prevention

The effectiveness of tamoxifen in preventing the recurrence of breast cancer in women with early disease led to the hypothesis that it may also be effective in preventing breast cancer in healthy women who are at high risk of developing the disease. To test this possibility, several clinical trials were conducted, including the Breast Cancer Prevention Trial, which was the largest of these studies and included a total of 13,388 women at high risk of developing breast cancer. The results of this trial, conducted from 1992-1997, showed that five years of daily tamoxifen (20 mg) treatment reduced the incidence of invasive and non-invasive breast cancers by 49% and 50%, respectively, compared to a placebo. Among the tamoxifen-treated subjects, a total of 124 breast cancer cases (89 invasive and 35 non-invasive) out of 6,576 patients were observed. Out of 6,599 placebo-treated patients, 244 cases of breast cancer were seen (175 invasive and 69 non-invasive). Non-invasive breast cancers, e.g. lobular carcinoma in situ (LCIS) and ductal carcinoma in situ (DCIS), are confined within the breast lobules, where milk is produced, or within the ducts, which drain milk from the lobules to the nipple. Invasive breast cancers are those that are no longer confined to these areas and have begun to invade the surrounding tissue. With respect to the incidence of estrogen receptor-positive breast cancers, tamoxifen treatment resulted in a 69% reduction (5.02 cases per 1,000 women with placebo vs. 1.58 cases per 1,000 women with tamoxifen). No difference was seen in the incidence of estrogen receptor-negative breast cancers [2]. These results led to the 1998 FDA approval of tamoxifen for reducing the risk of breast cancer in women deemed to be at high risk. A 2003 combined analysis of all the tamoxifen breast cancer prevention studies conducted up to that time showed that the overall incidence of breast cancer was reduced by 38%, with a 48% reduction in the incidence of estrogen receptor-positive breast cancer [41]. Finally, in the Study of Tamoxifen and Raloxifene (STAR) discussed later in this Chapter, tamoxifen and raloxifene were found to be equally efficacious in preventing invasive breast cancer [9].

Toremifene for Breast Cancer Treatment

Toremifene is a SERM closely related to tamoxifen, differing by a single chlorine atom. The effects of toremifene in breast cancer have been studied extensively, and multiple Phase III clinical trials have demonstrated that toremifene and tamoxifen are equally effective in treating advanced breast cancer, with very similar side effects [3-7]. Toremifene received FDA approval for the treatment of metastatic breast cancer in postmenopausal women in 1997. Additional studies have evaluated the efficacy of toremifene as an adjuvant treatment for preventing the recurrence of breast cancer. In these studies, toremifene again proved to be equivalent to tamoxifen [42, 43]. The most recently reported large clinical trial comparing tamoxifen and toremifene for the adjuvant treatment of early stage breast cancer was the North American Fareston versus Tamoxifen Adjuvant (NAFTA) trial, which enrolled a total of 1,813 perimenopausal or postmenopausal women with hormone receptor-positive (estrogen and/or progesterone receptor) invasive breast cancer. In agreement with previous trials, the NAFTA study found that overall survival and disease-free survival of women treated with toremifene or tamoxifen were the same, with similar side effect profiles [44]. Further evidence supporting toremifene for the adjuvant treatment of breast cancer was found in a recent Phase III trial in Japanese women with early breast cancer treated with either tamoxifen or toremifene daily for two years. This smaller study found that five-year survival and disease-free survival were very similar, again demonstrating that toremifene is equivalent to tamoxifen when used as an adjuvant breast cancer treatment [45]. Given the close chemical relationship between tamoxifen and toremifene, the results of these studies come as no surprise. Toremifene, however, has still not been FDA approved in this treatment setting.

At one time it was believed that toremifene would have a superior side effect profile compared to tamoxifen, while maintaining equivalent treatment efficacy. Indeed, reducing the incidence of side effects seen with tamoxifen treatment, especially endometrial cancer, was one of the goals when toremifene was originally synthesized. Toremifene has been shown to have a lower genotoxic potential (ability to bind to DNA, which can result in the development of cancer) [46-50], but based on the available clinical data it still remains unclear whether toremifene has any distinct advantage over tamoxifen with respect to the risk of endometrial cancer. The latest analyses do show that the incidences of endometrial cancers and other side effects with toremifene treatment may be lower, but the difference is not statistically significant [51, 52]. Although toremifene may have a slightly reduced risk of endometrial cancer compared to tamoxifen, it has many of the same side effects and thus is not currently being considered for breast cancer prevention.

Raloxifene for Breast Cancer Prevention

Raloxifene was originally developed for the treatment of breast cancer in the 1980s, but when compared to tamoxifen in clinical trials, the results were disappointing [8]. Later research showing the benefits of SERMs in bone without the increased risk of breast cancer associated with hormone replacement therapy led to the successful development of raloxifene for the treatment and prevention of postmenopausal osteoporosis [53]. During the development of raloxifene for osteoporosis, results of the Multiple Outcomes of Raloxifene Evaluation (MORE) trial revealed that raloxifene may be useful for the prevention of breast cancer. The MORE trial showed that after three years of daily treatment with raloxifene, the incidence of invasive breast cancer was reduced by 76% compared to placebo-treated women (13 cases out of 5,129 women treated with raloxifene compared to 27 cases out of 2,576 women treated with placebo) [54]. After four years of treatment, the incidence of invasive breast cancer was still 72% lower in the women treated with raloxifene (22 cases with raloxifene compared to 39 cases with placebo) [55]. In the MORE trial, raloxifene was not associated with an increased risk of endometrial cancer [56], which is not surprising due to its neutral effects in the uterus. A four-year extension of the MORE trial, known as the Continuing Outcomes Relevant to Evista® (CORE) trial, was conducted to determine the effects of four additional years of raloxifene treatment on breast cancer prevention. Overall, the incidence of invasive breast cancer was reduced by 59% with raloxifene treatment (24 cases out of 3,510 women) compared to placebo (28 cases out of 1,703 women). Estrogen receptor-positive breast cancers were reduced by 66% with raloxifene in this study (15 cases out of 3,510 raloxifene-treated women compared to 21 cases out of 1,703 women treated with placebo). A combined analysis of the data from the MORE and CORE studies showed an overall reduction in invasive breast cancer of 66% in women taking raloxifene compared to placebo-treated women over the eight-year study period [57]. Given these positive results, it was decided that tamoxifen and raloxifene should be compared head-to-head for the prevention of breast cancer in women at high risk.

The Study of Tamoxifen and Raloxifene (STAR trial) mentioned earlier was a randomized, double-blind clinical trial comparing the effects of daily tamoxifen (20 mg) to raloxifene (60 mg) for five years on the incidence of invasive breast cancer and other diseases. A total of 19,747 postmenopausal women (9,872 assigned to tamoxifen treatment and 9,875 assigned to raloxifene treatment) at increased risk of breast cancer were enrolled. The results showed that there was no meaningful difference in the incidence of invasive breast cancer (163 cases for tamoxifen versus 168 cases for raloxifene); however, the incidence of non-invasive breast cancer was lower in the tamoxifen-treated women (57 cases) compared to those who were treated with raloxifene (80 cases), though this difference did not prove to be significant. No differences in the frequency of other cancers, heart disease or stroke were observed. While raloxifene treatment was associated with fewer cases of endometrial cancer (23 cases vs. 36 for tamoxifen) and blood clots, these differences also did not prove to be significant [9]. Additional follow-up continued to show fewer cases of endometrial cancer with raloxifene treatment, as would be expected based on the known effect of raloxifene in the uterus [58]. Overall, raloxifene proved to be equivalent to tamoxifen in reducing the incidence of invasive breast cancer and inferior to tamoxifen in reducing the incidence of non-invasive breast cancer, with a reduced incidence of endometrial cancers. Following the results of the STAR trial, in 2007 the FDA approved raloxifene for reducing the risk of invasive breast cancer in postmenopausal women with osteoporosis and in those who are at high risk of developing the disease.

Ospemifene for Breast Cancer Treatment and Prevention

Unlike tamoxifen, toremifene and raloxifene, ospemifene has not been extensively studied for its effects in breast cancer in clinical trials. While standard breast safety assessments were performed in the various clinical trials of ospemifene, the specific effects of ospemifene on breast cancer were not studied clinically because the focus of Phase III development was postmenopausal vulvar and vaginal atrophy. However, the effects of ospemifene in the prevention and treatment of breast cancer were studied extensively in multiple animal models, as discussed in Chapter 4. In a rat model where breast cancer was induced using a chemical carcinogen, ospemifene effectively prevented the development of new tumors and caused existing tumors to shrink [14]. Two separate studies in mice, one lasting 37 weeks and the other 52 weeks, where breast cancer was again induced using a chemical carcinogen, compared the breast cancer preventive effects of ospemifene to tamoxifen, which is FDA approved for prevention of breast cancer in postmenopausal women at high risk. In both of these studies, ospemifene effectively prevented the development of breast tumors, similar to tamoxifen [16]. In a different mouse model where two different types of human breast tumors were implanted, ospemifene effectively inhibited the growth of only those tumors dependent on estrogen for growth [15]. Additional studies were performed in mice where precancerous breast tissue that transforms into breast cancer in a predictable fashion was transplanted into host animals. Ospemifene once again proved to be just as effective as tamoxifen in preventing the development of breast tumors [13]. In a related mouse model where breast cancer develops spontaneously under the influence of a viral oncogene (a gene that causes cancer), ospemifene was found to significantly increase survival when used as either a treatment or a preventive agent [12]. For detailed discussions of these and other related studies, please refer to Chapter 4.

This extensive body of preclinical data strongly suggests that ospemifene acts as an antiestrogen in normal breast tissue and breast cancer, as would be expected based on the known effects of other SERMs, and that it is effective in preventing breast cancer, similar to tamoxifen. There are currently no data, clinical or otherwise, that suggest ospemifene poses any breast-related risks. While the FDA required that the ospemifene labeling contain a breast cancer warning against use in women with known or suspected breast cancer or who are at high risk of developing breast cancer, this is simply a precaution due to limited clinical data rather than any specific scientific finding. The clinical data that are available demonstrated a very good breast safety profile for ospemifene. In all of the Phase II and Phase III clinical trials of ospemifene, only two cases of breast cancer were observed, both of which occurred in placebo-treated patients [59-61]. Future clinical studies of ospemifene as a breast cancer chemopreventive agent are needed to address the potential utility of ospemifene in this treatment setting. In fact, a Phase IV clinical trial of ospemifene in postmenopausal women at high risk for the development of breast cancer is being considered. Furthermore, given the established efficacy of ospemifene in treating dyspareunia associated with vulvar and vaginal atrophy and the fact that both tamoxifen and raloxifene aggravate this condition [9, 62], ospemifene could potentially be used to prevent breast cancer while improving dyspareunia in postmenopausal women at high risk of developing breast cancer.

Conclusion

One of the most frequently asked questions about ospemifene among clinicians since the drug was approved in 2013 has been "What are the effects of ospemifene in the breast?" Other SERMs such as tamoxifen, toremifene and raloxifene have established roles in the treatment and/or prevention of breast cancer. This class of drugs is known to have antiestrogenic effects in breast tissue, which makes them effective in breast cancer, where they antagonize the growth-stimulating effects of estrogen. Ospemifene is also a SERM, and like the already approved members of this drug class, it has demonstrated antiestrogenic effects in the breast in extensive preclinical animal-based studies. In these studies, ospemifene and tamoxifen were equally effective in preventing breast cancer. Ospemifene, however, carries an FDA warning against its use in women with a history of breast cancer. This is a result of the fact that ospemifene was not specifically studied for its effects in the breast in clinical trials due to the focus on vulvar and vaginal atrophy, not because of any known risk. All data published to date, including from the Phase III clinical trials, indicates that ospemifene is antiestrogenic in the breast, and it is not associated with any breast-related safety concerns. Additional clinical trials are needed to demonstrate whether ospemifene use in breast cancer patients is safe and whether it is effective for the prevention of breast cancer.

Problems with sexual dysfunction as a result of vulvar and vaginal atrophy symptoms in breast cancer survivors is a major quality of life issue now that increasing numbers of women are surviving breast cancer. The toxic effects of chemotherapy in the ovaries lead to early menopause in younger breast cancer patients, and hormonal therapy with aromatase inhibitors in estrogen-dependent cancer exacerbates symptoms of vaginal dryness and dyspareunia resulting in an already common problem among healthy postmenopausal women becoming even worse in breast cancer survivors. For women with hormone-dependent breast cancer, systemic estrogen-based menopausa hormone therapy cannot be used to alleviate vulvar and vaginal atrophy symptoms due to breast cancer risk, thus limiting treatment options for these women. While low-dose, short-course vaginal estrogen can be effective in these patients if non-hormonal remedies are inadequate, safety data are still quite limited. Should ospemifene be proven safe for breast cancer patients in future clinical trials, a valuable new, and much needed, treatment option for vulvar and vaginal atrophy in these patients would become available. Compared to tamoxifen and raloxifene, ospemifene could potentially offer an advantage in that it would improve symptoms of vulvar and vaginal atrophy while being equally effective for breast cancer prevention. It is our opinion, based on many years of research, that ospemifene will ultimately be proven safe for the treatment of vulvar and vaginal atrophy in breast cancer patients and for the prevention of breast cancer in postmenopausal women at high risk.

References

[1]   Siegel, R., Ma, J., Zou, Z., Jemal, A. (2014). Cancer statistics, 2014. *CA Cancer J Clin*, *64(1)*, 9-29.

[2]   Fisher, B., Costantino, J. P., Wickerham, D. L., Redmond, C. K., Kavanah, M., Cronin, W. M., et al. (1998). Tamoxifen for prevention of breast cancer: report of the National Surgical Adjuvant Breast and Bowel Project P-1 Study. *J Natl Cancer Inst*, *90(18)*, 1371-1388.

[3]   Gershanovich, M., Garin, A., Baltina, D., Kurvet, A., Kangas, L., Ellmen, J. (1997). A phase III comparison of two toremifene doses to tamoxifen in postmenopausal women with advanced breast cancer. Eastern European Study Group. *Breast Cancer Res Treat*, *45(3)*, 251-262.

[4]   Hayes, D. F., Van Zyl, J. A., Hacking, A., Goedhals, L., Bezwoda, W. R., Mailliard, J. A., et al. (1995). Randomized comparison of tamoxifen and two separate doses of toremifene in postmenopausal patients with metastatic breast cancer. *J Clin Oncol*, *13(10)*, 2556-2566.

[5]   Milla-Santos, A., Milla, L., Rallo, L., Solano, V. (2001). Phase III randomized trial of toremifene vs tamoxifen in hormonodependant advanced breast cancer. *Breast Cancer Res Treat*, *65(2)*, 119-124.

[6]   Pyrhonen, S., Ellmen, J., Vuorinen, J., Gershanovich, M., Tominaga, T., Kaufmann, M., et al. (1999). Meta-analysis of trials comparing toremifene with tamoxifen and factors predicting outcome of

antiestrogen therapy in postmenopausal women with breast cancer. *Breast Cancer Res Treat, 56(2)*, 133-143.

[7]   Pyrhonen, S., Valavaara, R., Modig, H., Pawlicki, M., Pienkowski, T., Gundersen, S., et al. (1997). Comparison of toremifene and tamoxifen in post-menopausal patients with advanced breast cancer: a randomized double-blind, the 'nordic' phase III study. *Br J Cancer, 76(2)*, 270-277.

[8]   Jordan, V. C. (2003). Antiestrogens and selective estrogen receptor modulators as multifunctional medicines. 1. Receptor interactions. *J Med Chem, 46(6)*, 883-908.

[9]   Vogel, V. G., Costantino, J. P., Wickerham, D. L., Cronin, W. M., Cecchini, R. S., Atkins, J. N., et al. (2006). Effects of tamoxifen vs raloxifene on the risk of developing invasive breast cancer and other disease outcomes: the NSABP Study of Tamoxifen and Raloxifene (STAR) P-2 trial. *JAMA, 295(23)*, 2727-2741.

[10] Soe, L. H., Wurz, G. T., Kao, C. J., Degregorio, M. W. (2013). Ospemifene for the treatment of dyspareunia associated with vulvar and vaginal atrophy: potential benefits in bone and breast. *Int J Womens Health, 5*, 605-611.

[11] Wurz, G. T., Soe, L. H., Degregorio, M. W. (2013). Ospemifene, vulvovaginal atrophy, and breast cancer. *Maturitas, 74(3)*, 220-225.

[12] Burich, R. A., Mehta, N. R., Wurz, G. T., McCall, J. L., Greenberg, B. E., Bell, K. E., et al. (2012). Ospemifene and 4-hydroxyospemifene effectively prevent and treat breast cancer in the MTag.Tg transgenic mouse model. *Menopause, 19(1)*, 96-103.

[13] Namba, R., Young, L. J., Maglione, J. E., McGoldrick, E. T., Liu, S., Wurz, G. T., et al. (2005). Selective estrogen receptor modulators inhibit growth and progression of premalignant lesions in a mouse model of ductal carcinoma in situ. *Breast Cancer Res, 7(6)*, R881-889.

[14] Qu, Q., Zheng, H., Dahllund, J., Laine, A., Cockcroft, N., Peng, Z., et al. (2000). Selective estrogenic effects of a novel triphenylethylene compound, FC1271a, on bone, cholesterol level, and reproductive tissues in intact and ovariectomized rats. *Endocrinology, 141(2)*, 809-820.

[15] Taras, T. L., Wurz, G. T., DeGregorio, M. W. (2001). In vitro and in vivo biologic effects of Ospemifene (FC-1271a) in breast cancer. *J Steroid Biochem Mol Biol, 77(4-5)*, 271-279.

[16] Wurz, G. T., Read, K. C., Marchisano-Karpman, C., Gregg, J. P., Beckett, L. A., Yu, Q., et al. (2005). Ospemifene inhibits the growth of

dimethylbenzanthracene-induced mammary tumors in Sencar mice. *J Steroid Biochem Mol Biol, 97(3)*, 230-240.

[17] Arora, N. K., Gustafson, D. H., Hawkins, R. P., McTavish, F., Cella, D. F., Pingree, S., et al. (2001). Impact of surgery and chemotherapy on the quality of life of younger women with breast carcinoma: a prospective study. *Cancer, 92(5)*, 1288-1298.

[18] Burwell, S. R., Case, L. D., Kaelin, C., Avis, N. E. (2006). Sexual problems in younger women after breast cancer surgery. *J Clin Oncol, 24(18)*, 2815-2821.

[19] Knobf, M. T. (2006). The influence of endocrine effects of adjuvant therapy on quality of life outcomes in younger breast cancer survivors. *Oncologist, 11(2)*, 96-110.

[20] Baumgart, J., Nilsson, K., Evers, A. S., Kallak, T. K., Poromaa, I. S. (2013). Sexual dysfunction in women on adjuvant endocrine therapy after breast cancer. *Menopause, 20(2)*, 162-168.

[21] Cella, D., Fallowfield, L., Barker, P., Cuzick, J., Locker, G., Howell, A. (2006). Quality of life of postmenopausal women in the ATAC ("Arimidex", tamoxifen, alone or in combination) trial after completion of 5 years' adjuvant treatment for early breast cancer. *Breast Cancer Res Treat, 100(3)*, 273-284.

[22] Kwan, K. W., Chlebowski, R. T. (2009). Sexual dysfunction and aromatase inhibitor use in survivors of breast cancer. *Clin Breast Cancer, 9(4)*, 219-224.

[23] Whelan, T. J., Goss, P. E., Ingle, J. N., Pater, J. L., Tu, D., Pritchard, K., et al. (2005). Assessment of quality of life in MA.17: a randomized, placebo-controlled trial of letrozole after 5 years of tamoxifen in postmenopausal women. *J Clin Oncol, 23(28)*, 6931-6940.

[24] Whelan, T. J., Pritchard, K. I. (2006). Managing patients on endocrine therapy: focus on quality-of-life issues. *Clin Cancer Res, 12(3 Pt 2)*, 1056s-1060s.

[25] Rosenberg, S. M., Partridge, A. H. (2013). Premature menopause in young breast cancer: effects on quality of life and treatment interventions. *J Thorac Dis, 5(Suppl 1)*, S55-61.

[26] Torino, F., Barnabei, A., De Vecchis, L., Appetecchia, M., Strigari, L., Corsello, S. M. (2012). Recognizing menopause in women with amenorrhea induced by cytotoxic chemotherapy for endocrine-responsive early breast cancer. *Endocr Relat Cancer, 19(2)*, R21-33.

[27] Ganz, P. A., Coscarelli, A., Fred, C., Kahn, B., Polinsky, M. L., Petersen, L. (1996). Breast cancer survivors: psychosocial concerns and quality of life. *Breast Cancer Res Treat, 38(2)*, 183-199.

[28] Ganz, P. A., Desmond, K. A., Belin, T. R., Meyerowitz, B. E., Rowland, J. H. (1999). Predictors of sexual health in women after a breast cancer diagnosis. *J Clin Oncol, 17(8)*, 2371-2380.

[29] Pinto, A. C., de Azambuja, E. (2011). Improving quality of life after breast cancer: dealing with symptoms. *Maturitas, 70(4)*, 343-348.

[30] Green, L. M. Addressing Sexual Concerns in Breast Cancer Patients and Survivors. Oncology Nursing News. 2014:22-24.

[31] Goodwin, P. J., Ennis, M., Pritchard, K. I., Trudeau, M., Hood, N. (1999). Risk of menopause during the first year after breast cancer diagnosis. *J Clin Oncol, 17(8)*, 2365-2370.

[32] Meirow, D. (2000). Reproduction post-chemotherapy in young cancer patients. *Mol Cell Endocrinol, 169(1-2)*, 123-131.

[33] NAMS (2013). Management of symptomatic vulvovaginal atrophy: 2013 position statement of The North American Menopause Society. *Menopause, 20(9)*, 888-902.

[34] Greenblatt, R. B., Barfield, W. E., Jungck, E. C., Ray, A. W. (1961). Induction of ovulation with MRL/41. Preliminary report. *JAMA, 178*, 101-104.

[35] Morello, K. C., Wurz, G. T., DeGregorio, M. W. (2002). SERMs: current status and future trends. *Crit Rev Oncol Hematol, 43(1)*, 63-76.

[36] Osborne, C. K. (1998). Tamoxifen in the treatment of breast cancer. *N Engl J Med, 339(22)*, 1609-1618.

[37] Saez, R. A., Osborne, C. K. *Breast Cancer* Current Clinical Oncology 1. B. J. Kennedy, editor. New York: Alan R. Liss; 1989. 163-172 p.

[38] Clarke, M., Collins, R., Davies, C., Godwin, J., Gray, R., Peto, R. (1998). Tamoxifen for early breast cancer: an overview of the randomised trials. Early Breast Cancer Trialists' Collaborative Group. *Lancet, 351(9114)*, 1451-1467.

[39] Davies, C., Godwin, J., Gray, R., Clarke, M., Cutter, D., Darby, S., et al. (2011). Relevance of breast cancer hormone receptors and other factors to the efficacy of adjuvant tamoxifen: patient-level meta-analysis of randomised trials. *Lancet, 378(9793)*, 771-784.

[40] Davies, C., Pan, H., Godwin, J., Gray, R., Arriagada, R., Raina, V., et al. (2013). Long-term effects of continuing adjuvant tamoxifen to 10 years versus stopping at 5 years after diagnosis of oestrogen receptor-positive breast cancer: ATLAS, a randomised trial. *Lancet, 381(9869)*, 805-816.

[41] Cuzick, J., Powles, T., Veronesi, U., Forbes, J., Edwards, R., Ashley, S., et al. (2003). Overview of the main outcomes in breast-cancer prevention trials. *Lancet, 361(9354)*, 296-300.

[42] Holli, K. (2002). Tamoxifen versus toremifene in the adjuvant treatment of breast cancer. *Eur J Cancer, 38 Suppl 6*, S37-38.

[43] Holli, K., Valavaara, R., Blanco, G., Kataja, V., Hietanen, P., Flander, M., et al. (2000). Safety and efficacy results of a randomized trial comparing adjuvant toremifene and tamoxifen in postmenopausal patients with node-positive breast cancer. Finnish Breast Cancer Group. *J Clin Oncol, 18(20)*, 3487-3494.

[44] Lewis, J. D., Chagpar, A. B., Shaughnessy, E. A., Nurko, J., McMasters, K., Edwards, M. J. (2010). Excellent outcomes with adjuvant toremifene or tamoxifen in early stage breast cancer. *Cancer, 116(10)*, 2307-2315.

[45] Kimura, M., Tominaga, T., Kimijima, I., Takatsuka, Y., Takashima, S., Nomura, Y., et al. (2014). Phase III randomized trial of toremifene versus tamoxifen for Japanese postmenopausal patients with early breast cancer. *Breast Cancer, 21(3)*, 275-283.

[46] Hard, G. C., Iatropoulos, M. J., Jordan, K., Radi, L., Kaltenberg, O. P., Imondi, A. R., et al. (1993). Major difference in the hepatocarcinogenicity and DNA adduct forming ability between toremifene and tamoxifen in female Crl:CD(BR) rats. *Cancer Res, 53(19)*, 4534-4541.

[47] Hellmann-Blumberg, U., Cartner, M. G., Wurz, G. T., DeGregorio, M. W. (1998). Intrinsic reactivity of tamoxifen and toremifene metabolites with DNA. *Breast Cancer Res Treat, 50(2)*, 135-141.

[48] Hellmann-Blumberg, U., Taras, T. L., Wurz, G. T., DeGregorio, M. W. (2000). Genotoxic effects of the novel mixed antiestrogen FC-1271a in comparison to tamoxifen and toremifene. *Breast Cancer Res Treat, 60(1)*, 63-70.

[49] Karlsson, S., Hirsimaki, Y., Mantyla, E., Nieminen, L., Kangas, L., Hirsimaki, P., et al. (1996). A two-year dietary carcinogenicity study of the antiestrogen toremifene in Sprague-Dawley rats. *Drug Chem Toxicol, 19(4)*, 245-266.

[50] White, I. N., de Matteis, F., Davies, A., Smith, L. L., Crofton-Sleigh, C., Venitt, S., et al. (1992). Genotoxic potential of tamoxifen and analogues in female Fischer F344/n rats, DBA/2 and C57BL/6 mice and in human MCL-5 cells. *Carcinogenesis, 13(12)*, 2197-2203.

[51] Gu, R., Jia, W., Zeng, Y., Rao, N., Hu, Y., Li, S., et al. (2012). A comparison of survival outcomes and side effects of toremifene or

tamoxifen therapy in premenopausal estrogen and progesterone receptor positive breast cancer patients: a retrospective cohort study. *BMC Cancer, 12*, 161.

[52] Harvey, H. A., Kimura, M., Hajba, A. (2006). Toremifene: an evaluation of its safety profile. *Breast, 15(2)*, 142-157.

[53] Delmas, P. D., Bjarnason, N. H., Mitlak, B. H., Ravoux, A. C., Shah, A. S., Huster, W. J., et al. (1997). Effects of raloxifene on bone mineral density, serum cholesterol concentrations, and uterine endometrium in postmenopausal women. *N Engl J Med, 337(23)*, 1641-1647.

[54] Cummings, S. R., Eckert, S., Krueger, K. A., Grady, D., Powles, T. J., Cauley, J. A., et al. (1999). The effect of raloxifene on risk of breast cancer in postmenopausal women: results from the MORE randomized trial. Multiple Outcomes of Raloxifene Evaluation. *JAMA, 281(23)*, 2189-2197.

[55] Cauley, J. A., Norton, L., Lippman, M. E., Eckert, S., Krueger, K. A., Purdie, D. W., et al. (2001). Continued breast cancer risk reduction in postmenopausal women treated with raloxifene: 4-year results from the MORE trial. Multiple outcomes of raloxifene evaluation. *Breast Cancer Res Treat, 65(2)*, 125-134.

[56] Grady, D., Ettinger, B., Moscarelli, E., Plouffe, L., Jr., Sarkar, S., Ciaccia, A., et al. (2004). Safety and adverse effects associated with raloxifene: multiple outcomes of raloxifene evaluation. *Obstet Gynecol, 104(4)*, 837-844.

[57] Martino, S., Cauley, J. A., Barrett-Connor, E., Powles, T. J., Mershon, J., Disch, D., et al. (2004). Continuing outcomes relevant to Evista: breast cancer incidence in postmenopausal osteoporotic women in a randomized trial of raloxifene. *J Natl Cancer Inst, 96(23)*, 1751-1761.

[58] Runowicz, C. D., Costantino, J. P., Wickerham, D. L., Cecchini, R. S., Cronin, W. M., Ford, L. G., et al. (2011). Gynecologic conditions in participants in the NSABP breast cancer prevention study of tamoxifen and raloxifene (STAR). *Am J Obstet Gynecol, 205(6)*, 535 e531-535.

[59] Goldstein, S. R., Bachmann, G. A., Koninckx, P. R., Lin, V. H., Portman, D. J., Ylikorkala, O. (2014). Ospemifene 12-month safety and efficacy in postmenopausal women with vulvar and vaginal atrophy. *Climacteric, 17(2)*, 173-182.

[60] Simon, J., Portman, D., Mabey, R. G., Jr. (2014). Long-term safety of ospemifene (52-week extension) in the treatment of vulvar and vaginal atrophy in hysterectomized postmenopausal women. *Maturitas, 77(3)*, 274-281.

[61] Simon, J. A., Lin, V. H., Radovich, C., Bachmann, G. A. (2013). One-year long-term safety extension study of ospemifene for the treatment of vulvar and vaginal atrophy in postmenopausal women with a uterus. *Menopause, 20(4)*, 418-427.

[62] Land, S. R., Wickerham, D. L., Costantino, J. P., Ritter, M. W., Vogel, V. G., Lee, M., et al. (2006). Patient-reported symptoms and quality of life during treatment with tamoxifen or raloxifene for breast cancer prevention: the NSABP Study of Tamoxifen and Raloxifene (STAR) P-2 trial. *JAMA, 295(23)*, 2742-2751.

Glossary of Terms

Adipose Tissue
Fat tissue.

Adjuvant
A therapy administered following an initial treatment; for example, tamoxifen is given following breast cancer surgery to prevent recurrence of the disease.

Agonist
A drug that exerts an effect initiated through a receptor (compare to antagonist).

Ambient Temperature
Environmental temperature.

Amenorrhea
Cessation of the menstrual cycle.

Anastrozole
An aromatase inhibitor used in the adjuvant treatment of breast cancer that acts by inhibiting the activity of the enzyme aromatase, which produces estrogen in the body.

Ancillary Study
A smaller study related to a larger main study.

Androgen
A generic term for any of several male sex hormones.

Antagonist
A drug that inhibits the initiation of drug activity through a receptor (compare to agonist).

Antiestrogenic Effects
Effects that oppose the activity of estrogen.

Aromatase Inhibitor
Any of a class of breast cancer drugs that act by inhibiting the action of the enzyme aromatase, resulting in extremely low levels of circulating estrogen.

Arterial Calcification
Calcium deposits in the arteries.

Asymptomatic
Lack of symptoms.

Atrophic Vaginitis
Thinning and inflammation of the vagina.

Autonomic Nervous System
Part of the nervous system that helps control blood pressure, blood flow and heart rate, among many other physiologically important functions.

Baseline Rate
Rate established at the beginning of a clinical trial, for example.

Baseline Result
A result or measurement established at the beginning of a clinical trial, for example.

Bazedoxifene
A selective estrogen receptor modulator (SERM) that is used for the treatment of postmenopausal osteoporosis.

Bioavailability
A measure of the quantity of a drug available to the body to exert pharmacological effects.

Bioequivalence
Having the same or similar biological effect.

Body Mass Index (BMI)
The ratio of one's body weight expressed in kilograms to the square of one's height expressed in meters.

Bone Mineral Density
A measurement of the density of calcium and other minerals in the bone. This measurement is used to estimate the strength of bone.

Bone Resorption
The breakdown of loss of bone.

Bone Turnover
Also known as bone remodeling. The combined process of bone formation and bone resorption.

Capillary Beds
The smallest blood vessels in the body. They deliver oxygen and nutrients to the various tissues in the body.

Cardiovascular
Related to the heart and blood vessels.

Cardiovascular Disease (CVD)
Disease related to the heart and blood vessels.

Carotid Intima Media Thickness
Thickness of the carotid (neck) arteries.

Center for Drug Evaluation and Research (CDER)
Center for Drug Evaluation and Research. Branch of the U.S. Food and Drug Administration that deals with the evaluation and approval of drugs.

Central Nervous System (CNS)
Part of the nervous system comprising the brain and spinal cord.

Chemoprevention
The prevention of a disease or condition using a drug.

Chemotherapy
The treatment of cancer using drugs.

Clonidine
A medication for hypertension (high blood pressure). It blocks the release of the neurotransmitter norepinephrine (noradrenaline).

Cognitive Function
Brain function related to memory and thoughts.

Confounding Factor
Something that interferes or influences.

Conjugated Estrogens
A mixture of different forms of estrogen, as found in the commercial pharmaceutical product Premarin®.

Contraindication
A pre-existing condition that could worsen when a treatment is administered for an unrelated health issue.

Coronary Atherosclerosis
Hardening of the heart (coronary) arteries.

Coronary Heart Disease (CHD)
A narrowing of the small blood vessels that supply blood and oxygen to the heart. Also called coronary artery disease.

Cross-sectional Survey
A survey done across a vast population at the same time.

Deep Vein Thrombosis
A blood clot that forms in a deep vein such as in the lower leg.

Dementia
General mental deterioration characterized by disorientation and impaired memory, judgment and intellect; for example, Alzheimer's disease.

Drug Efficacy Study Implementation (DESI)
Drug Efficacy Study Implementation. An FDA program designed to evaluate the efficacy of drugs that had been approved prior to 1962.

Diethylstilbestrol (DES)
A synthetic form of estrogen.

Dyspareunia
Painful sexual intercourse.

Efficacy
A measure of effectiveness, as of a drug.

Endometrial Hyperplasia
Excessive proliferation of the cells of the inner lining of the uterus (endometrium), leading to endometrial thickening.

Endometrium
The inner lining of the uterus.

Estradiol
The most potent form of the estrogenic female sex hormones.

Estrogen
Generic term for any of several related estrogenic female sex hormones.

Estrogen Receptor
A protein where estrogen binds to produce a stimulatory effect.

Estrogen Receptor Agonist/antagonist
A chemical compound, e.g. a SERM, that can bind to the estrogen receptor, producing either a stimulatory (agonist) or inhibitory (antagonist) effect depending on the tissue.

Estrogen Replacement Therapy (ERT)
The administration of estrogen after menopause to replace the diminished natural production of the hormone.

Fat Mass
Measurement of fat tissue in the body.

First-line Treatment
Method or treatment used as the first approach.

Flushing
A sensation of warmth that appears suddenly, as in a hot flush or flash associated with menopause.

Follicle-Stimulating Hormone (FSH)
Hormone secreted from the pituitary gland that regulates follicular maturation and estrogen production by the ovaries in females and the production of sperm by the testes in males.

Generic Drug
A non-branded medication that is bioequivalent to the brand name form of the medication.

Half-life
A measure of the length of time required for the elimination of half of the circulating quantity of a drug from the body.

Heart Palpitations
A sensation that the heart is pounding or racing; a common menopausal symptom.

Heart Estrogen/progestin Replacement Study (HERS)
Heart Estrogen/progestin Replacement Study. The first large clinical trial that was designed specifically to assess whether the risk of coronary heart disease events in postmenopausal women with known coronary disease is reduced with the use of estrogen plus progestin hormone therapy.

Hormone Replacement Therapy (HRT)
A treatment consisting of an estrogen and a progestin for the alleviation of menopausal symptoms. This term is also used generically for any hormone treatment for menopausal symptoms.

Hot Flash
A sudden sensation of warmth experienced as a symptom of menopause; also called hot flush.

4-Hydroxyospemifene
The main metabolite of Osphena™ (ospemifene).

Hyperplasia
An abnormal increase in the number of cells in a tissue or organ causing part or all of the tissue or organ to become enlarged.

Hypothalamus
Part of the brain that controls body temperature, among many other critical functions.

Hysterectomy
Surgical removal of the uterus.

Incontinence
Inability to control urination.

Intermediate Cells
Cells in the middle layer of the vaginal epithelium.

Investigational New Drug (IND)
A new experimental drug that has received FDA approval to enter clinical trials. Also the application for approval to enter clinical trials.

Lean Mass
Muscle mass in the body.

Letrozole
An aromatase inhibitor used in the adjuvant treatment of breast cancer that acts by inhibiting the activity of the enzyme aromatase, which produces estrogen in the body.

Longitudinal Survey
A study that follows a group of subjects over a long period of time.

Mare
Term for a female horse.

Medroxyprogesterone Acetate (MPA)
A synthetic progestin commonly used as part of hormone replacement therapy. Also used in birth control preparations.

Menopausal Status
A determination, based on menstruation and sex hormone levels, of whether a woman is premenopausal, perimenopausal or postmenopausal.

Menopausal Transition
The transition from premenopause to perimenopause to postmenopause.

Menopause
The natural stage of a woman's life marked by loss of ovarian production of the female sex hormone estrogen, resulting in permanent cessation of menstruation.

Meta-analysis
The analysis of the combined results of several clinical trials.

Metabolite
A product of the enzymatic breakdown of a drug substance.

Monotherapy
Treatment with a single compound.

Most Bothersome Symptom (MBS)
The symptom of vulvar and vaginal atrophy, e.g. dyspareunia and vaginal dryness, which a postmenopausal woman perceives as being the most bothersome.

North American Menopause Society (NAMS)
North American Menopause Society. Founded in 1989, NAMS is North America's leading nonprofit organization dedicated to promoting the health and quality of life of all women during midlife and beyond through an understanding of menopause and healthy aging.

Neuron
A nerve cell.

Neurotransmitter
Chemical messenger used as a means of communication between neurons.

New Drug Application (NDA)
An application for the approval of a new drug by the FDA. This application is the final step in the drug development process and is based on all of the research conducted on a particular drug, from preclinical animal studies all the way through Phase III clinical trials.

Non-topical
A treatment that is not administered through the skin.

Norepinephrine
A catecholamine neurotransmitter, also known as noradrenaline, that causes vasoconstriction (narrowing) of blood vessels, thereby increasing blood pressure. In the brain, norepinephrine plays an important role in alertness and arousal.

Observational Study
A type of clinical study in which individuals are observed and certain outcomes are measured without any attempt to affect them. This type of study does not involve the administration of study medications.

Osphena™
Trade name for the SERM ospemifene.

Osteoblast
A type of bone cell involved in the formation of new bone.

Osteoclast
A type of bone cell involved in the resorption or destruction of existing bone.

Osteoporosis
A condition characterized by weak, porous, brittle bones that are at an increased risk of fracture.

Ovarian Insufficiency
Insufficient production of female sex hormones by the ovaries.

Ovarin
Primitive treatment for menopausal symptoms developed in the late 19th century that was derived from the ovaries of cows.

Parabasal Cells
The innermost layer of cells in the vaginal epithelium.

Paroxetine
Generic name for Paxil[®], an antidepressant agent in the drug class known as selective serotonin reuptake inhibitors (SSRIs).

Perimenopause
Period between premenopause and postmenopause.

Peripheral Vascular Reactivity
Reactivity (constriction and relaxation) of the peripheral blood vessels. Increased peripheral vascular reactivity is associated with hot flashes, a common menopausal symptom.

Peripheral Vasculature
Blood vessels in the body's periphery.

Pharmacokinetics
Measurements of the absorption, distribution, metabolism and excretion of a drug substance in the body.

Physiological
Relating to normal anatomical function.

Placebo Effect
A psychological effect that occurs when a person believes they are receiving a beneficial medication.

Polymorphism
A variation in the DNA sequence of a gene that leads to minute changes in the encoded protein.

Postmenopause
Time period after menopause.

Premarin®
Trade name for conjugated equine estrogens.

Premenstrual Symptoms
Symptoms developing prior to the menstrual period.

Progesterone
A female sex hormone that plays a prominent role during pregnancy. Progesterone is used as part of hormone replacement therapy to protect the endometrium from the potentially carcinogenic effects of estrogen.

Progestin
A progesterone-like drug, e.g. medroxyprogesterone acetate (MPA) commonly used in HRT, which simulates the activity of the female sex hormone progesterone.

Pulmonary Embolism
A blood clot that becomes lodged in and restricts the flow of blood through blood vessels, e.g. the pulmonary artery, in the lungs.

Raloxifene
A SERM that has been FDA approved for the treatment and prevention of postmenopausal osteoporosis and for reducing the risk of breast cancer in women at high risk.

Reuptake
Reabsorption or retrieval, as of a neurotransmitter.

Selective Estrogen Receptor Modulator (SERM)
A chemical compound that possesses both estrogenic and antiestrogenic effects depending on the tissue. For example, the breast cancer drug tamoxifen opposes the effects of estrogen in the breast but has estrogen-like effects in the bone.

Serotonin
A neurotransmitter that plays a key role in regulating mood, blood flow, and blood pressure.

Sleep Parameters
Measurements of sleep quality.

Study of Women's health Across the Nation (SWAN)
Study of Women's health Across the Nation. One of the largest and most ethnically diverse longitudinal studies of the menopausal transition that followed over 3,000 women for over 10 years.

Stroke
A sudden impairment in the delivery of blood to a part of the brain as a result of a blood clot (thrombotic or ischemic stroke) or a burst blood vessel (hemorrhagic stroke).

Subcutaneous Fat
Fat beneath the skin.

Superficial Cells
Cells in the uppermost layer of the vaginal epithelium.

Symptomatic
Related to symptoms.

Systemic
Across the system.

Tamoxifen
A SERM used in the treatment of all stages of breast cancer, and for reducing the risk of breast cancer in postmenopausal women at high risk. Tamoxifen was the first clinically useful SERM.

Testosterone
The principal male sex hormone.

Thermoregulation
Control of body temperature.

Toremifene
A SERM in the same chemical class as tamoxifen that is used for the treatment of metastatic breast cancer. Toremifene is also the parent drug of ospemifene.

Triglycerides
Fats circulating in the blood.

Unopposed estrogen
Taking estrogen for the treatment of menopausal symptoms without the use of a progestin.

Urethral Musculature
Muscles surrounding the opening of the urethra, which carries urine from the bladder out of the body.

Urinary Tract
The system composed of the kidneys, ureters (which carry urine from the kidneys to the bladder), bladder and urethra.

Urogenital Health
The health of the urinary tract and genitalia.

Vaginal Epithelium
Lining of the vagina.

Vaginal Maturation Index (VMI)

Vaginal Maturation Index. An index which takes into account the ratios of parabasal cells, intermediate cells, and superficial cells of the vaginal epithelium. The VMI is used to assess the efficacy of treatments for vulvar and vaginal atrophy.

Vaginal pH

Measurement of the acidity and basicity of the vagina.

Vaginal Vault

Top of the vagina.

Vasoconstriction

Narrowing of the blood vessels.

Vasomotor Symptoms (VMS)

Symptoms commonly experienced during the menopausal transition. Vasomotor symptoms principally comprise hot flashes and night sweats.

Venlafaxine

An antidepressant drug in the class of selective serotonin and norepinephrine reuptake inhibitors (SNRI).

Vulvar and Vaginal Atrophy (VVA)

Thinning of the lining of the vulva and vagina.

Women's Health Initiative (WHI)

A major women's health project funded by the National Institutes of Health (NIH) to study the major health effects of hormone replacement therapy in postmenopausal women aged 50-79. The initiative was principally comprised of two large clinical trials, one that studied estrogen alone in hysterectomized postmenopausal women and one that studied estrogen plus progestin in postmenopausal women with a uterus.

Women's Health Initiative Memory Study (WHIMS)

An ancillary study to the WHI studies that evaluated the effects of estrogen alone and estrogen plus progestin on cognition in postmenopausal women aged 65-79.

Yohimbine

A chemical that increases the release of the neurotransmitter norepinephrine.

Index

C

Postmenopause, 177
post-transplant, 80
potential benefits, 53, 89, 106, 160
precocious puberty, 120
pregnancy, 4, 31, 32, 43, 177
Premarin® Vaginal Cream, 28, 29, 30, 31,
32, 33, 34, 35, 36, 46, 110, 111, 113,
115, 116, 117, 118, 120, 121, 123
Prempro®, 52
primary tumor, 152
prodrugs, 72
progesterone, 2, 3, 4, 73, 83, 152, 154, 164,
177
Progestin(s), 37, 40, 42, 47, 51, 59, 64, 67,
111, 113, 126, 177
prolactin, 77
proliferation, 77, 80, 86, 87, 106, 171
protection, 8, 45, 60, 75, 105
proteins, 73, 86
Prozac®, 6
public health, ix, 30
pulmonary embolism, 57, 111, 113, 119

Q

quality of life, x, 1, 2, 5, 7, 11, 13, 16, 17,
19, 23, 45, 93, 108, 128, 150, 158, 161,
162, 165, 175

R

race, 7, 10, 21
Raloxifene, 34, 71, 79, 87, 131, 133, 144,
148, 155, 156, 164, 177
randomized controlled clinical trials, 49, 54
rash, 120
reactions, 6, 116, 117, 119, 120, 122, 124,
125
reactivity, 5, 20, 105, 163, 176
receptors, 21, 23, 27, 33, 70, 73, 104, 152,
162
recurrence, 150, 152, 153, 154, 167
regulations, 27, 30, 36, 41, 44, 116
regulatory requirements, 44

response, 4, 26, 79, 80, 81, 82, 117, 138,
152
risk factor(s), 7, 8, 22, 53
risk profile, 30, 33, 34, 109, 117, 123
risks, ix, x, 3, 10, 28, 29, 30, 32, 33, 34, 35,
36, 40, 41, 51, 55, 56, 58, 63, 65, 104,
109, 110, 111, 114, 115, 116, 118, 123,
141, 148, 149, 151, 153, 157
Royal Marsden breast cancer prevention
trial, 132

S

Selective estrogen Menopause And
Response to Therapy (SMART), 136
selective estrogen receptor
modulator(SERM), 17, 34, 37, 58, 69,
70, 102, 103, 105, 106, 107, 115, 123,
127, 129, 142, 143, 145, 147, 148, 160,
168, 178
selective serotonin reuptake inhibitor, 46,
176
selectivity, 106
sensation, 2, 4, 5, 6, 7, 12, 20, 21, 172, 173,
178, 180
serum, 23, 71, 72, 73, 83, 84, 86, 87, 88,
102, 134, 135, 136, 138, 140, 142, 164
sex, 1, 2, 3, 8, 16, 23, 31, 42, 150, 168, 171,
174, 176, 177, 179
sex hormones, 3, 8, 42, 168, 171, 176
sex steroid, 23
sexual activity, 92, 99
sexual desire, 4, 16, 20
Sexual dysfunction, 161
sexual health, 16, 19, 162
sexual intercourse, ix, 1, 2, 15, 42, 69, 150,
171
sexual problems, 150
side effects, ix, x, 17, 27, 29, 30, 31, 32, 34,
35, 44, 48, 55, 57, 58, 69, 85, 87, 90, 92,
94, 99, 103, 109, 110, 115, 116, 129,
130, 131, 137, 153, 154, 163
skin, 6, 9, 21, 43, 74, 78, 120, 147, 175, 178
skin cancer, 147
sleep disturbance, 7, 12

W

Y